Lingzhi
From Mystery to Science

Zhi-Bin Lin, M.D.
Professor of Pharmacology
Peking University Health Science Center
Beijing, China

English editor: Linda Gray Huang

Peking University Medical Press

Lingzhi From Mystery to Science, First Edition 2009

ISBN 978-7-81116

Copyright ©c 2009 by Peking University Medical Press

Published by Peking University Medical Press, 38 Xueyuan Road, Beijing 100191, China

Home Page:http://www.pumpress.com.cn

E-mail:booksale@bjmu.edu.cn

Printed by Beijing Jiaxinda Art Press Co., Ltd.

Distributed by Beijing Issuing House, New China Book Store (38.00)

Printed in the People's Republic of China

Supported by

Medical Publishing Foundation of

Peking University Health Science Center

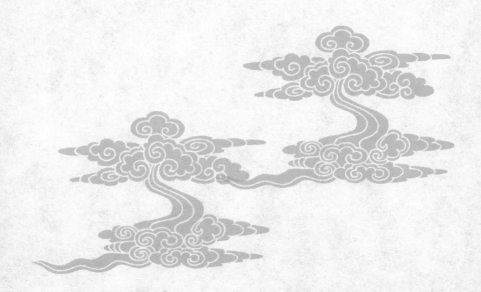

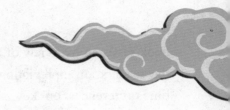

Preface

Lingzhi (*Ganoderma lucidum*) is historically a treasured herbal material in China. It is becoming well-known all over the world in recent years. The Chinese traditional medicine's classic, *Shennong Materia Medica*, regards Lingzhi as being of a "supremely exquisite" quality with tonic and longevity effects. Over the years, fables and legends adored Lingzhi with a patina of mystery as a "heavenly herb" that connotes auspiciousness, blissfulness and happiness.

Professor Zhi-Bin Lin, a distinguished pharmacologist, has devoted a life-long study on Lingzhi. With his extraordinary insights on the culture, pharmacology, physiology, chemistry and clinical applications associated with Lingzhi, Prof. Lin presents in this book the scientific understanding of the herb's beneficial functions on human immune, nervous, endocrine and cardiovascular systems. Thus, Lingzhi has been applied as an adjuvant treatment for cancer patients, and also a food supplement to improve general health and wellness.

Lingzhi from Mystery to Science is written based on actual research and clinical findings. Prof. Lin explains the complex theories in commonly understandable language. In addition, this book gives an overview of the classic literature and legends to allow the readers an appreciation of the "Lingzhi culture". At the same time, references on key scientific studies relevant to the various functions as explained in separate headings are listed for those who need further information. The readers can become familiar with Lingzhi's efficacy and the basic aspects concerning the diseases, such as chronic bronchitis, hyperlipidemia, hypertension, diabetes, hepatitis, tumors, dermal and urological diseases, sub-health and aging, as well as its nutraceutical applications. Peeling off the mystical patina, *Lingshi from Mystery to Science* unveils the truth of Lingzhi that may help in the public's better understanding of such a wonderful material and usher in the author's ultimate purpose of promoting the health and well-being of mankind.

Professor Chen Keji, M.D.
Academician, Chinese Academy of Sciences
Honorary Chairman, Chinese Association of Integrative Medicines
Beijing, May 2009

Foreword

A Chinese herb medicine, the fruiting body of Lingzhi, *Ganoderma lucidum*, has been used as a folk remedy in China for thousands of years, as reported in *Shenong Materia Medica*. Increasing research in the modern times elucidates numerous pharmacological effects of Lingzhi, including immunomodulating and anti-tumor, anti-atherosclerosis, lipid-lowering, hypoglycemic, liver-protective, anti-oxidative, free radical scavenging and anti-aging activities. Recent clinical studies in China also prove that Lingzhi can be used to treat bronchitis, arteriosclerosis, neurasthenia and insomnia, hepatitis, diabetes, cancers and aging.

Nowadays, both in China and abroad, extensive research and industrial development has lead Lingzhi and a vast variety of its products to be widely applied for the prevention and cure of diseases, as well as for the improvement of health and general well-being. However, along with the commercialization, quality of and advertisement for the products has become a concern. The product quality varies greatly, and the claims on the efficacy and functions are frequently untrue, or exaggerated to say the least. To confront such undesirable outcomes, perhaps, the best way is to provide consumers with the scientific information on Lingzhi in plain and easily understandable language.

With that, the idea of writing a popular science book on Lingzhi was born. In preparation, I reviewed volumes of available promotional materials on Lingzhi. Indeed, I discovered that while the commercial literature full of misleading descriptions, the popular science publications were largely lacking rigorous scientific evidence. A year ago, the book, *Lingzhi: From Mystery to Science*, in Chinese was published. To reach a wider readership, this English version has been translated from the Chinese edition. In particular, some of the clinical trials were conducted in the past under very different circumstances from today. The in vitro tests can hardly be duplicated nowadays. Consequently, the existing information is invaluable for anyone who is interested in the study of Lingzhi. Most of the clinical reports were written in Chinese when they first appeared. Through this publication, it is hoped that researchers and consumers worldwide may benefit.

In the book, original reports on the systematic clinical studies, rather than individual cases, relating to Lingzhi's medicinal efficacy are presented for the discussion. In Chapters 3, 14 and 15 comprehensive information is presented on Lingzhi product' s quality, usage and processing technologies. During my decades of research on Lingzhi, I have become deeply interested in the ancient Chinese literature, traditional culture and the philosophy associated with Lingzhi. Lingzhi's spiritual and mystical image is ingrained and permeated in the people, culture and tradition. It comes with its graceful appearance and magic efficacy. Thus, in Chapter 1 and 2, the historical legends and evidence, which has evolved into Lingzhi's symbolic meaning of happiness and longevity, are briefed to reflect my earnest hope for the health and well-being of all.

This book refers much of its scientific research results from what is in *Modern Research of Ganoderma lucidum, 3rd Edition* (by Zhi-Bin Lin, Peking University Medical Press, Beijing, 2007). For the detailed information, therefore, readers are advised to refer to that publication. Other references that are directly cited are listed immediately following the text in this book.

My sincere thanks to Associate Professor X.L. Zhu, M.D. for her assistance, and to my colleagues, L. Lu, M.D.; X; Wang, M.D.; L Tie, M.D.; Mr. J.S. Gao; Ms. J.Z. Zhang; Ms. X.R. Shi; Ms. Y.S. Li; Ms. M. Li and Ms. Y.Q. Ou, for their contribution in translating the first draft from Chinese into English, and Prof. Frank Huang and Ms. Linda G. Huang for final editing. Without their help, it would not have been possible to complete this book. Lastly, I must pay tribute to the grant provided for the publication by Peking University Health Science Center.

Zhi-Bin Lin, M.D.
Professor of Pharmacology
Peking University Health Science Center

Contents

Chapter 3

Chapter 4

Chapter 5

Chapter 6

Chapter 7

Chapter 8

Chapter 9

Chapter 10

Chapter 11

Chapter 12

Chapter 13

Chapter 14

Chapter 15

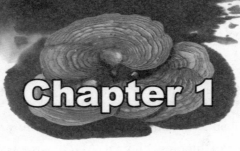

Chapter 1

Mystery and Culture of Lingzhi

Author's prompt: Historically, Lingzhi (*Ganoderma lucidum*) has been viewed as a magic herb as well as an auspicious symbol by Chinese. It is, therefore, also known as "Ruizhi" , "Shenzhi" and "Xiancao," with the meaning of good fortune and mysterious power. Numerous myths and poems mentioning people's love, worshipping and beliefs on Lingzhi can be found in Chinese literature since ancient time. Taoism played an important role in promoting Lingzhi for either medical purposes or otherwise. To date, many Chinese idioms, such as "Ji Xiang Ru Yi" (good fortune and happiness), "Ci Fu Jia Xiang" (bestow blessing and happiness), "Zeng Tian Shou Kao" (blessed with longevity), "Guo Tai Ming An" (country is prosperous and people live in peace), continue to be used by the people reflecting the ingrained "Lingzhi culture".

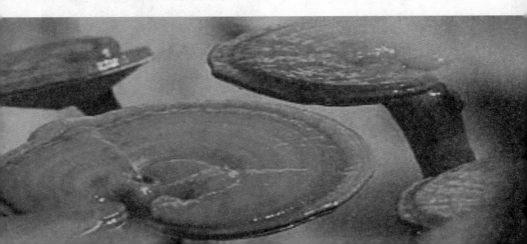

Lingzhi in myths

More than two thousands years ago, there was already evidence of Chinese worshipping Lingzhi. Myths associated with this magic plant can be found in history.

In the *Book of Mountains and Seas* of the Warring States Period (476–221B.C.), the young daughter of Emperor Yan, Yaoji, was mystified that she turned into the herb, Yaocao (Grass of Yao), after she died. A poet from Chu, Song Yu engaged her in the fairy tale love story with a god. The myth eventually made Yaoji the origin of Lingzhi.

In the *Legend of the White Snake*, the heroine White Snake went alone to Mt. Emei to steal the celestial herb (i.e., Lingzhi) in order to save her husband's life. She overcame all sorts of hardships and finally moved the heart of the God, who let her have the magical herb that revived her husband from dead. The love story has become the subject of countless novels, dramas, movies and posters in China (Fig. 1-1).

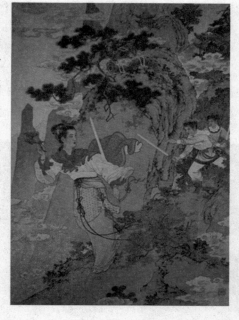

Fig. 1-1 Poster of the White Snake stealing Lingzhi

Lingzhi in ancient poems

Lingzhi is the symbol of sanctity and goodness. It was a common motif in the Chinese literature in the past.

A famous poet from Chu, Qu Yuan described in his poem, *Nine Sons, Mountain Ghost*, a goddess longing for love. "Sanxiu" in the poem was another name for Lingzhi, which can be harvested more than once a year. The "Mountain Ghost", on the other hand, was the goddess who picked Lingzhi in Mt. Wu.

When Emperor Hanwudi officiated the sacrificial ritual, 70 young boys and girls would chant *The Song of Lingzhi* with the music. The lyric carried the messages of wishing for auspiciousness, good fortune and longevity.

In the Period of Three Kingdoms, poet Cao Zhi referred frequently to Lingzhi. For instance, in his well-known poem, *On Lingzhi*, he praised Lingzhi as creating the heaven and earth, the maroon herb growing along the bank of River Luo symbolized the prosperity of the nation and the glory of the god. In his *Praise of the Goddess Luo*, the poet depicted how graceful and beautiful the Goddess Luo was harvesting Lingzhi, and his admiration of

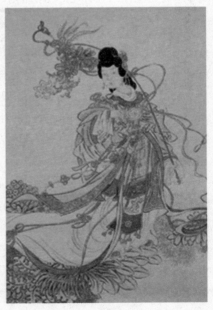

Fig. 1-2 Goddess Luo holding Lingzhi (Painting by Ren Xiong of Qing Dynasty)

3

the goddess (Fig. 1-2). In the *Flying Dragon*, he told a story of his encounter in the misty Mt. Tai with a Taoist monk on a white deer with a Lingzhi in his hand. It was from that man he learned the magic health benefits of Lingzhi.

In the *Singing Trip of a Han Dynasty* Yuefu-style poem, a similar story was told. The author met a god-like man with short hair and long ears riding a white deer, and was led to pick Lingzhi. At the legendary man's home, he was shown the tonic made from the health-improving, hair-color darkening, and life-prolonging effects of the reddish herb.

"Catholicon" according to Taoism

The "Lingzhi culture" was greatly influenced by Taoism, the native religion in China. Taoism believes that living is most important and that human beings can be immortal by following the regimens and taking a certain magical herbs. *Bao Pu Zi* written by Ge Hong presented the theory suggesting that a person could learn to become immortal. It even included stories of such occurrences by taking Lingzhi.

The ancient Taoist theory considered Lingzhi as the best among the catholicons, and by consuming Langzhi, one would never grow old or die. Therefore, Lingzhi acquired the names, such as Shenzhi (heavenly herb) and Xiancao (magic grass), and became mystified. In the book of *Ten Continents in the World*, Lingzhi grew everywhere in the fairy land. Gods fed on it to gain immortality. In the Jin Dynasty, Wang Jia's *Picking Up the Lost* and in the Tan Dynasty, Dai Fu's *The Vast Oddities*, 12,000 varieties of Lingzhi were said to be cultivated on acres of land in Mt. Kunlun by the gods. Ge Hong, in his *Legend of the Gods*, the beautiful goddess, Magu, pursued Taoism at Mt. Guyu and lived on the Panlai Isle. She brewed the Lingzhi wine specifically for the Queen's birthday. This picture of Magu holding the wine, a child raising a birthday peach-shaped cake, an old man with a cup and a crane with Lingzhi in its mouth has become a popular folk art for birthday celebration with the wishes of fortune and longevity (Fig. 1-3).

Most of the famous Taoists in history, including Ge Hong, Lu Xiu-Jing, Tao Hong-Jing and Sun Si-Miao, saw the importance of Lingzhi studies. They influenced greatly in promoting the Lingzhi culture in China. In pursuing immortality, the Taoists enriched the knowledge on the herb and led to the evolution of the Taoist medical practice, which emphasize health and well-being.

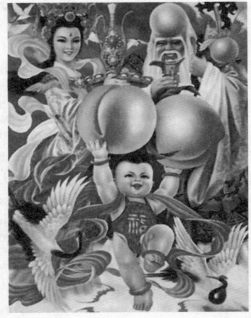

For their philosophy as well as a lack of scientific knowledge, the Taoists' understanding of Lingzhi was not only limited but also mostly superstitious. The term, "zhi," used by them referred to many other kinds of fungi. It even included the mythical and imaginary herb. The religious connection was criticized by the medical profession in China and impeded the progress of

Fig. 1-3 Poster of Magu for birthday wishes

Lingzhi's applications and true understanding.

 ## Auspicious symbol for Chinese

Since the Han Dynasty, Confucius scholars gave Lingzhi the names of "fortune herb" or "fortune grass". They considered the circular lines on top of Lingzhi cap an auspicious symbol or fortunate halos. Gradually, the lucky charm characteristic of Lingzhi became a unique component in Chinese culture.

Han History on Emperor Wu recorded the growth of Lingzhi in the palace that initiated a royal parole as the Emperor saw it as an auspicious sign. And, the lyric of a song said, "An herb with nine stems was harvested from the House of Qi; Children were excited and placed on the alter; Its thriving growth brought out the inspirational spirit of the auspicious herb." In fact, the rotten wood in the palace allowed the fungus to sprout and grow. The officers made up the story to please the Emperor, and he believed it.

In the Song Dynasty, Wang An-shi wrote about how people were forced by the government officers to search for Lingzhi in his *In Praise of Lingzhi Pavillion*. Thousands of farmers and villagers went into mountains, on cliffs, in valleys and the wilderness to look for the herb. *The History of Song Dynasty* indicated, during the 25 years ruled by Emperor Zhenzong, Lingzhi was attributed 116 times. Emperor Shi zong of the Ming Dynasty piled up Lingzhi brought to him in the palace to form a "Lingzhi hill". To collect such a great quantity of Lingzhi from all over the country with few available means of transportation had to be a paramount task.

On the enormous Ming Dynasty mural, *Making Tribute to the King*, in Shanxi, the expression of a court lady with the gift of Lingzhi in her hands shows the ritualistic of the tribute-giving process at the time. That is a precious art masterpiece (Fig. 1-4).

For Chinese, Lingzhi and its derivative, Ruyi (literally, as one wishes, Fig.1-5), have been the symbol for luck, fortune, longevity, peace and prosperity. This widely believed in and deeply affects the people and culture to date. Images of Ling-zhi, and the "fortunate clouds" derived from it, can be found on palaces, temples, ancient buil-dings, clothing, embroidery,

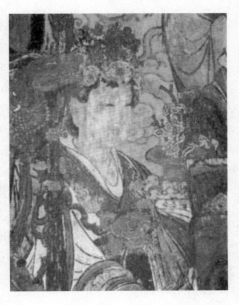

Fig. 1-4 Portion of the gigantic mural, *Making Tribute to the King*, in Shanxi

paintings, sculptures, china and excavated archaeological relics. For example, they are on the pole infront of the Tiananmen Square (Fig. 1-6), on the ceiling of the Qinian Hall at the Temple of Heaven, and

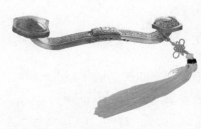

Fig. 1-5 A colored glaze handi-craft of Ruyi

on the royal passage leading to the Main Hall at the Forbidden City. There are carved Lingzhi bonsai on the fences at the Forbidden City, the Ancient Ministry of Education Building and the Confucius Temple, the graphic design on the base of the stone tablet at the Confucius Temple, as well as the wood-carving of Ling-

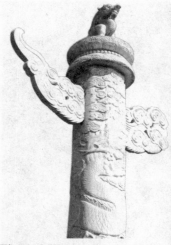

Fig. 1-6 "Fortunate clouds" design on the pole at Tiananmen Square

zhi bonsi before the Sakyamuni statue in Yonghe Lamasery. These give the evidence of how Chinese worshiped Lingzhi in the old time.

The silk painting by Emperor Qianlong of the Qing Dynasty (Fig. 1-7), a collection at the Palace Museum in Taipei, shows a vase with pine branches, camellia and plum blossom. And, on its side there are persimmon, lilies and Lingzhi. This is a typical painting reflecting the wish for good luck and fortune.

Guo Mo-Ruo's poem on Lingzhi

In 1958, a farmer found a Lingzhi shaped like a dear horn in Mt. Huang. When the Chinese renown poet, Guo Mo-Ruo, heard of it, he wrote a poem that was published in *The People's Daily*(December 28, 1958):

Lingzhi on the Lion Apex, more than 200 meters high.

Who picked it? An old farmer named Yang.

With a height of 49 cm, many marks on the stem.

Roots are shiny and bright, with colors of white, green and golden.

Red, like coral reflecting light, of the most precious variety.

Seen as an auspicious sign is no surprise, for they are everywhere nowadays.

Finding this Lingzhi has reasons, as the mysterious Qilin's appearance.

All living beings are liberated, socialism celebrates spring forever.

In the poem, the location, shape, size, color and type of the Lingzhi found were described. Guo might have derived the descriptions from Ge Hong's book, in which Lingzhi was said to be like meat, attached to large rocks, with head and tail and a living organism; the red ones with color of coral, the white ones that of the fat, the black ones lacquer, the green ones peacock feather, the yellow ones gold; and, they were all shiny and hard like ice. The authors showed their admirations of Lingzhi. Guo also used the symbol to wish prosperity of the nation.

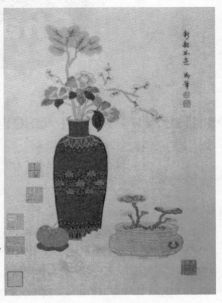

Fig. 1-7 Silk painting by Emperor Qianlong of Qing Dynasty

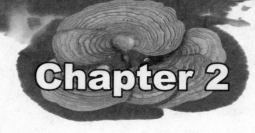

Chapter 2

Lingzhi As Described in *Shennong Materia Medica*

Author's Prompt: *Shennong Materia Medica* and many other written records in early Chinese history began to study, discuss and report the scientific aspects of Lingzhi in respect to its categorization, habitat, bionomics, herbal nature, medication, etc. They have been frequently referred to in literature and used for further research and applications. At the same time, incorrect or unsubstantiated information continues to be weeded out and updated.

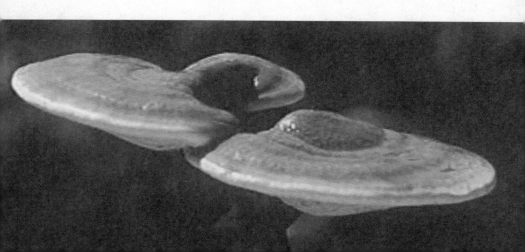

Shennong Materia Medica on Lingzhi

The earliest history of Lingzhi's discovery and application by Chinese can be dated back 2000 years to the Spring and Autumn Period (770−476 B.C.) and Warring States Period (475−221 B.C.). In Zhou Dynasty (1112−221 B.C.), *Scholars Discussing Medicines* reported the fungal growth on rotted wood. It is the first known record of Lingzhi in the world.

Written in ca. 100 B.C., *Shennong Materia Medica* has the earliest pharmaceutical mention of Lingzhi. Shennong (God of Agriculture, Fig. 2-1) is a mythic figure. The book's real author is not known. Nonetheless, this monumental treatise listed 365 medicinal materials in 3 categories according to their medicinal and side effects on human. The highest graded materials were those with medicinal efficacies without known toxicity. Lingzhi (including Cizhi, Qingzhi, Huangzhi, Baizhi, Heizhi and Zizhi, which are red, blue, yellow, white, black and purple in color, respectively) was among the highest graded materials, based on the categorization.

Based on the Chinese medicinal theory of Yin and Yang and the 5- Elements, *Shennong Materia Medica* categorized Lingzhi according to their colors into Cizhi (or Danzhi), Heizhi (or Xuanzhi), Qingzhi (or Longzhi), Baizhi (or Yuzhi) and Huangzhi (or Jinzhi) as "Five Zhi," as well as Zizhi (or Muzhi). Detailed descriptions on their medicinal nature, sensory properties and medication were included in the book indicating that Cizhi was bitter in taste, mild in nature and non-toxic, and could be used for relieving chest congestion and improving memory; Heizhi was salty, mild and non-toxic, and could be used for renal problems and increasing awareness; Qingzhi was acidic, mild and

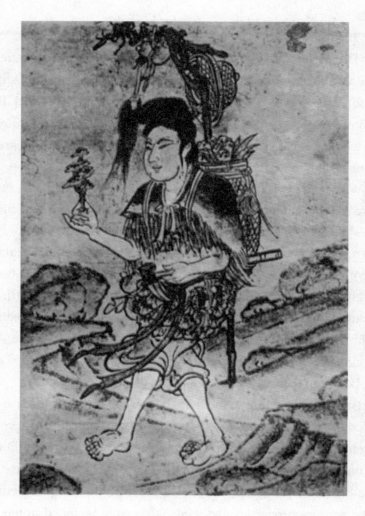

Fig. 2-1   A Liao Dynasty era painting on the wall of a wooden pagoda in Shanxi showing a barefooted man with a plump face and bared belly, covered himself with fur and leaves, shouldered a bamboo basket, held a Lingzhi and walked in a rocky mountain. Scholars believe that the man in the picture was Shennong, the God of Agriculture.

nontoxic, and could be used to improve eyesight and liver functions; Baizhi was pungent, mild and non-toxic, and could be used to cure coughs and ailments of the lungs; Huangzhi was sweet, mild and non-toxic, and could be used to rid of heart, spleen and stomach illnesses; and, Zizhi was sweet, warm(mild) and non-toxic, and could be used to help hard-hearing and arthritis. In addition, it emphasized that all 6 kinds of Lingzhi could be applied long term to facilitate health, well-being and longevity. Such information on Lingzhi is considered the classic reference for the Chinese medicine and has been quoted frequently in the literatures to date.

 ## Scientific understanding on Lingzhi by scholars in early years

Even in the early history, Chinese scholars already exhibited substantial understanding on the biological characteristics of Lingzhi. In *Scholars*, the author observed that "Zhi grows above the rotten soil". In *Speaking of Balance*, Wang Chong of the Eastern Han Dynasty pointed out that "Lingzhi grows from soils with balanced conditions". And, Tao Hong-Jing stated that "Zizhi, of the appearance of mushrooms, grows from the rotted tree trunks." It is evident that in the ancient time, it was already known that Lingzhi requires rotten soil or decaying wood to grow.

As mentioned in the last chapter, *Magic Medicines* described Lingzhi as organisms with red coral, white fat, lacquer black, peacock green or golden yellow color, were bright and transparent like ice, in the sizes ranging from 5 kg to 1.5 kg. The color, appearance and weight of the Lingzhi fruiting body were rather precisely recorded.

Furthermore, the mention of such things as "growing without

flower are Zhi mushrooms" (from *Liji Notes*), "rootless plant of Ling-zhi" (from *Erya Notes*), "three crops a year of Lingzhi" (from the *Compendium of Materia Medica*) and "all 6 kinds of Lingzhi can be harvested in June and August in a year" (from the *Compendium of Materia Medica*), show that the facts of these fungi are different from higher plants. The facts that Lingzhi have no roots, stem and leaf differentiation, do not flower and can be harvested several times in a year were known among the people working with Lingzhi in the early times.

The fact that Lingzhi can be used for medicinal purposes or as food were also recorded in Chinese history. For example, Wang Chong of the Eastern Han Dynasty stated in *Speaking of Balance*, "Lingzhi produces 3 crops in a year. Including it in diet can result in longevity as it is god's food." The legendary Chinese doctor, Li Shi-Zhen, pointed out that, "Lingzhi has been harvested around the year for the gods. It is safe for consumption and should be considered as a vegetable." Tao Hong-Jing believed that, "One may eat Lingzhi without a concern of dosage." On the other hand, Su Jing thoughtfully indicated that, "Ling-zhi is so rare. It is difficult to find them. How can anyone expect to have it continuously for a long period of time?" Therefore, it is apparent that Chinese at the time already knew Lingzhi's health benefits and anti-aging effects. However, the limited availability of the naturally grown Lingzhi prevented widespread applications.

Criticism on misinformation regarding Lingzhi in the old time

Misinformation on Lingzhi exists in many Chinese medical literatures, including the classic *Shennong Materia Medica*. Criticisms by scholars were found. Su Jing disagreed with the association of 5 Ling-

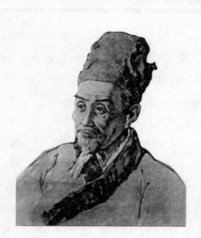

Li Shi-Zhen
(1518–1593 A.D.)

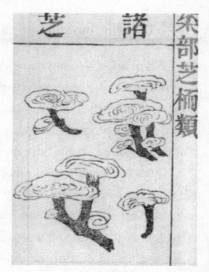

Fig. 2-2 Illustration of Lingzhi in the *Compendium of Materia Medica* by Li Shi-Zhen

zhi with their growing areas: "The red Lingzhi was found not limited to Mt. Huo, the black not limited to Mt. Heng, the blue Lingzhi not limited to Mt. Tai, the white Lingzhi not limited to Mt. Hua, and the yellow Lingzhi not limited to Mt. Song." Su's observation is correct, as we know these varieties of wild Lingzhi can indeed be found in most parts of China. In the *Compendium of Materia Medica*, Li Shi-Zhen re-classified Lingzhi according to the 5 colors and 5 "elements." His different viewpoints included that "Lingzhi of different colors logically taste differently, but their taste may not necessarily be directly correlated to their color." More importantly, Li criticized the superstitious aspects associated with Lingzhi. He also showed an accurate picture of Lingzhi in his book (Fig. 2-2).

Current understanding of the six kinds of Lingzhi

When ancient scholars referred to "Zhi group", they often meant mushrooms, not necessarily Lingzhi. In 1990s, mycologist Zhao Ji-Ding and others used a modern biological classification system on the "6 Zhi" described in *Shennong Materia Medica*. The results concluded that these "6 Zhi" are not all Lingzhi.

Qingzhi: Qingzhi (blue Lingzhi) could be a species similar to Yunzhi (*Coriolus versicolor or Polystictus versicolor*). The cap of Yunzhi has circular permutations and is covered by blue, dark blue, yellowish-brown, brown, white and black fine hairs. Its shiny, feather-like pattern is similar to the description of Qingzhi by Ge Hong: "green like the feathers of a peacock." But, Yunzhi does not belong to the *Ganoderma genus*.

Cizhi: Cizhi (red Lingzhi) is Lingzhi (*Ganoderma lucidum*) or Songsha Lingzhi (*Ganoderma tsugae*). Its red or purple, lacquer-like glossy cap does match the old description by Ge Hong: "red like coral..." It is scientifically proven that these two species have medicinal value. Cizhi is listed in the "*Pharmacopoeia of the Peoples Republic of China (Part1)*"as a traditional Chinese medicine(TCM), while Songshan Lingzhi has been approved by the Chinese government for health food production.

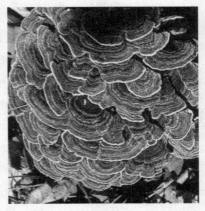

Fig 2-3 Yunzhi (From: Mao Xiao-Lan, *Large Fungi in China*. Henan Science and Technology Press, 2000.)

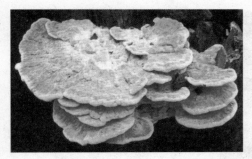

Fig. 2-4 Liuhuangjun (From: Mao Xiao-Lan, *Large Fungi in China*. Henan Science and Technology Press, 2000.)

Huangzhi: Based on the description Ge Hong put forth in *Bao Pu Zi* for Huang-zhi, it is speculated to be the Liuhuangjun (sulfur mush-room in Chinese, Fig. 2-4) (*Laetiporus sulphureus or Tyromyces sulphureus*). This fungus has a reddish-orange, yellowish-orange or light yellow colored cap, and turns whitish-yellow after dried. It is edible when young and tender. Adenine, betaine and other alkaloids have been isolated from this fungus. However, its medicinal value is still under investigation.

Baizhi: Ge Hong described Baizhi "white as fat". The possible fungus species is thought to be Kubaiti (pharmaceutical shelf fungus or pharmaceutical quinine fungus, *Fomitopsis officinalis*). The cap of Kubaiti is white to grayish-white in color. The flesh is grayish-white with meat-like texture, and becomes cheese-like with a bitter taste in the later stages of growth. It is used for invigorating the stomach functions or as a diaphoretic in Chinese medical practices.

Heizhi: The "black as lacquer" description of Heizhi's color leads to the proposal of identifying it as the Jiazhi (pseudo-lingzhi) or Wuzhi (black lingzhi) (*Amauroderma rugosum*). As the names imply, the fungus' cap is dull brown, dark brown, blackish-brown to black in color. It has a black, long stem. It is also possible that Heizhi is actu-ally Heibing duokong mushroom (*Polyporus melanopus*), which is white at the early stage and turns gradually to tea brown with a black

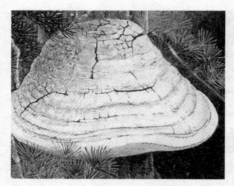

Fig. 2-5 Kubaiti (From: Mao Xiao-Lan, *Large Fungi in China*. Henan Science and Technology Press, 2000.)

brown to black stem.

Zizhi: It is most likely the Purple Lingzhi (*Ganoderma sinense*). Its cap is purplish-brown, purplish-black or black in color with lacquer-like gloss. The medicinal efficacy of Purple Lingzhi has been documented and it is listed in the *Pharmacopoeia of the Peoples Republic of China (Part 1)* as a Chinese herb medicine.

 Interpretation of *Shennong Materia Medica* using the traditional Chinese and Western medicine principles

Shennong Materia Medica was the summation of the experiences gained by the ancient Chinese medical practitioners. The legend of the God of Agriculture, who tasted a hundred herbs and encountered 70 poisonous ones in a day, gives the discovery process a vivid picture. Likewise, the medicinal information on Lingzhi shown in *Shennong Materia Medica* was obtained through practices. By integrating the traditional Chinese and the Western medicine principles to interpret the ancient literature, we may gain a better understanding of the facts regarding Lingzhi and thus help usher in further applications for the benefit of mankind.

To date, research on Lingzhi by combining the traditional Chinese medicine (TCM) and the Western medical science has already shown significant advances. For example, the pharmacological studies proved that Lingzhi can strengthen the heart, prevent myocardial ischemia, improve myocardial micro-circulation and regulate blood lipids, etc. Lingzhi is currently used in treatment of hyperlipidemia and coronary heart disease, possibly relating to the belief the

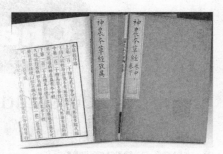

Shennong Materia Medica

"heart boosting" and "chest congestion relieving" effects recorded in the TCM books. Similarly, those "nerve soothing", "soul calming", "brain nourishing" and "memory improving" qualities of Lingzhi stated in *Shennong Materia Medica* seem to correspond to the functions, such as sedating and memory-improving, as well as treatments for neurasthenia and insomnia, as used in the modern medical research. The anti-oxidation and free radical scavenging ability of Lingzhi relates directly to anti-aging and health promoting effect for the middle aged and senior citizens. This is coincident to the statements in *Shennong Materia Medica*: "Lingzhi, when consumed regularly and for a long period of time, can energize the body, and retard aging." While, the "strengthening the internal organs" and the "boosting energy" properties of Lingzhi indicated in this book involve even broader roles, including immunological regulation and invigoration of the vital organs, such as the heart, lung, liver and kidneys, etc. Base on the understanding, we can come to a conclusion on Lingzhi's medicinal efficacy and health benefits for human beings. It is through the ability of Lingzhi to regulate human nerve-endocrine-immunity system that smoothly functioning, highly adaptable and well-balanced physical conditions can be realized. And, therefore, our health and well-being can be assured.

Chapter 3

Understanding Lingzhi

Author's prompt: The growth phases of Lingzhi include the stages of spores, mycelium and fruiting body. The spores are minute, single-cell, reproductive organ of the fungus. After germination, mycelia are formed and the fruiting bodies developed. The fruiting body, or basidioma, is the umbrella-shaped fruit. From the time of the ancient book of *Shenong Materia Medica* to the current *Pharmacopoeia of the People's Republic of China*, the fruiting body has been referred to as "Lingzhi," not other parts of the fungus. Lingzhi is traditionally cultivated on logs. However, for ecological concerns, environmental-friendly and sustainable cultivation methods are now advocated. In fact, to assure products of high quality, using reliable strains and following organic farming practice in cultivating Lingzhi are necessary and prudent for the business.

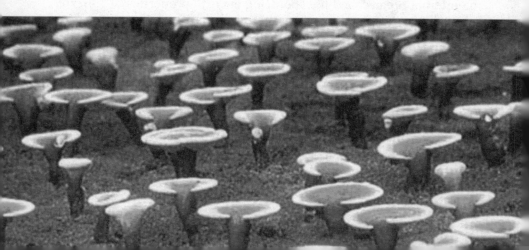

Lingzhi fruiting body — a Chinese medicine

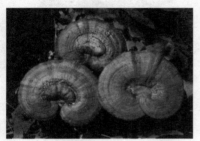

Fig. 3-1 *G. lucidum*

What is Lingzhi? It should not be a difficult question to answer. However, exaggerated or misleading advertisement and claims complicated the issue. Some distorted information led consumers to be lieve that the spores is the "essence" of Lingzhi. So, truthfully and scientifically, what is Lingzhi after all?

According to the biological classification, Lingzhi is an fungi belonging to Eumycota, Basidiomycetes, Polyporaceae, *Ganoderma* genus. Only its fruiting body is what has been referred to as "Lingzhi," historically and worldwide. The *Compendium of Materia Medica* stated that the Chinese word, "zhi," was originally derived from the shape of the Lingzhi fruiting body. As a plant (rather than an animal), a " grass" portion was added to create the Chinese character that we know today.

The genus *Ganoderma* includes sub genera *Ganoderma* (sect. *Ganoderma* and *Phaeo-nema*), *Trachyderma* and *Elfvingia*. There are 75 species in genus *Ganoderma* that can be found in China. But, only a few, such as *G. lucidum* (Leyss.ex.Fr) Karst (Fig. 3-1), *G. sinense* Zhao, Xu et Zhang (Fig. 3-2), *G. tsugae* Murr (Fig. 3-3) and *G. capense* (Lio-yd) Teng (Fig. 3-4), can be used for medicinal

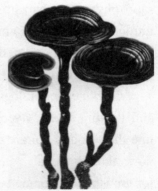

Fig. 3-2 *G. sinense*

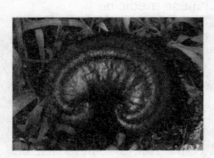

Fig. 3-3   *G. tsugae*

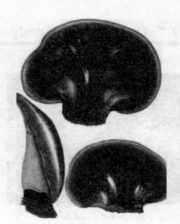

Fig. 3-4   *G. capense*

or food purposes. And, only the fruiting bodies of *G. lucidum* and *G. sinense* are considered medicinal materials by the *Pharmacopoeia of the People's Republic of China (2005 ed.Part I)*.

 ## Life cycle of Lingzhi

Like all fungi or mushrooms, Lingzhi has no chlorophyll, and cannot synthesize carbohydrates via photosynthesis. It is by means of saprophytism or parasitism, Lingzhi acquires its needed carbon and nitrogen from other organic sources. This way of sustaining life is called heterotrophy, as opposed to morphosis. It differentiates Lingzhi and the higher, green plants.

Grown either on logs or culture media, Lingzhi consists of mycelia and fruiting body. Mycelium is the white hyphae, which penetrates into the wood or culture medium. It is extremely powerful in breaking down those materials with various enzymes in order to extract nutrients for growth. The fruiting body grows above the log or medium and relea-ses basidiospore (spores) when ripens.

Merely a minute portion of the spores released from the fruiting body would land on adequate places (e.g., dead or decaying wood) and germinate into mycelium. Under appropriate conditions, the "primary" mycelia will grow into the "secondary" and "tertiary" mycelia, and eventually, fruiting body. In the late phase of a fruiting body, basidium is formed and basidiospores produced (Fig. 3-5).

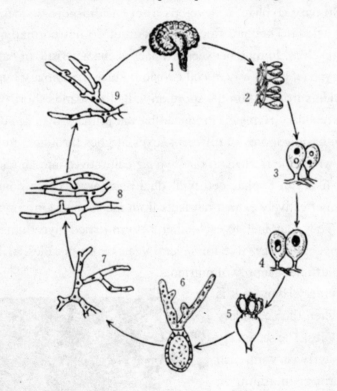

Fig. 3-5 Life cycle of Lingzhi: 1. Fruiting body; 2. Enlarged partial hymenium; 3. Basidium; 4. Internal matching in basidium; 5. Basidiospores released from basidium; 6. Germinating basidiospore; 7. Monocaryon hyphae; 8. Plasmogamy between two monocaryon hyphaes; 9. Dikaryon hyphae.

Morphological characteristics of hyphae, fruiting body and spores

Mycelium   Covered with white crystalline material, mycelium has a fuzzy, hairy appearance. Three types of hyphaes make up the mycelium. They are:

(A) Primary Hyphae: It develops from basidiospore. Its cell has only one nucleus. They are fine filaments, but do not normally join among themselves. Joining between hyphaes is characteristic of basidiomycetes hyphae. It is a way of cell division. Since the primary hyphae draws nutrients from within the spore only, its life span is short.

(B) Secondary Hyphae: Produced by the primary hyphaes developed from basidiospores of different sexes, it goes through a unique process in which the nucleus in one hyphae cell moves into another to become a dikaryon hyphae cell with duel nucleuses. The secondary hyphaes can effectively extract nutrients from media, and form mycelia (Fig. 3-6). They may lock to each other to form joined mycelium. The resultant mycelium may live for several years, even decades, as long as there is sufficient supply of nutrients.

(C) Tertiary Hyphae: It is the stage when the secondary hyphae matures. The secondary hyphaes may twist with each other to form primordium on the surface of the medium. Then, the primordium turns into tertiary hyphae, which grows into fruiting body. Structurally,

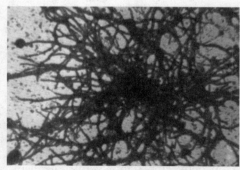

Fig. 3-6 Mycelia of Lingzhi

the tertiary hyphae is quite different from the secondary hyphae. The former have less voids in-between, and they also begin to show tissue and organ differentiations, such as stem and cap.

Fruiting Body   The fruiting body of Lingzhi is a reddish-purple or reddish-brown mushroom shaped like an umbrella. When young, its texture is like meat, but turns woody upon maturation. The fruiting body has a cap (pileus) on top of the stem (stipe).

The stem is irregular and cylindrical, and not always straight. If two stems touch each other, they will likely merge into a thicker one. The stem is mauve in color, darker on the side facing the sunlight than the shady side. Its diameter and length vary with the environmental and nutritional conditions. When sufficient nutrients are available, thicker stems will result, or vise versa. When area is well ventilated, the stem tends to grow short. If the oxygen supply is limited and carbon dioxide concentration high, the stem will end up tall and slender.

The internal structures of the cap and the stem are similar, except that the stem does not have a tube layer:

(A) Crust Layer: It is made up of three sub-layers: (1) The outermost layer is composed of many closely arranged thick hyphaes. The hyphae tips line up grid-like in parallel, and perpendicular to the cap. Its cell wall is thick and filled with resin and pigments giving the color and glossy appearance of the cap. (2) The middle layer is made up of interwoven thick-walled hyphaes. Inside the hyphaes, the reddish-brown resin produces the color of the cap. A mauve colored cap indicates a healthy fruiting body with a thick middle layer. Otherwise, the color is light and middle layer thin. (3) The inner layer is formed by interwoven hyphaes with no resin or pigments inside. The cell wall is thick. This layer is a transition stage from the crust to become the flesh.

(B) Flesh Layer: It is constituted by interwoven hyphaes that contain large vacuoles. These hyphaes pack together loosely with many voids in-between resulting in the characteristic cork-like texture of this layer.

(C) Tube Layer: This layer has many parallel-arranged tubes of hyphases. The end of the hyphae expands to an eggplant-like basidium. The basidium has a thin cell wall, dense cytoplasm and two nucleuses. As the fruiting body grows, the basidium gradually matures and the two nucleuses fuse to form one by the process of karyogamy. Then, twice, the fused nucleus divides into four sub-nucleuses through mitosis. At the same time, four small enations arise from the free end of the basidium and extend to form sterigmas. An oval basidiospore is generated at the top of the cone-shaped sterigma. When basidiospore matures, a vacuole between basidiospore and sterigma begins to absorb water until ruptures. The basidiospore is ejected through the tube cavity into the air when the vacuole bursts by virtue of the mechanical force. This produces the phenomenon of spore spreading.

Basidiospore   Under the microscope, the usually single-cell basidiospore is oval in shape and brown in color. It is Lingzhi's reproductive body, approximately 8–12 micrometers by 5–7 micrometers in dimension. It is covered by the double-layered cell-wall (sporoderm). The outer layer of the wall is smooth, colorless and transparent. Observed under an electron microscope, pits and holes can be seen on the outer wall (Fig. 3-7). The inner layer is dark brown with small enations. Inside the wall, the cavity is filled with thick cytoplasm, in which nest a nucleus and a yellow to bright yellowish-green oil droplet.

 ## Cultivation of Lingzhi for its fruiting bodies

To cultivate Lingzhi, hyphaes are isolated from the fruiting body, inoculated onto a log or culture medium, and allowed to grow into fruiting bodies under appropriate conditions. There are two major stages in cultivating Lingzhi, namely, (a) selection and propagation of strains suitable for the cultivation, and (b) cultivation of the fruiting body.

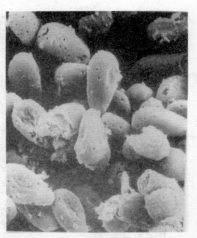

Fig. 3-7 Electron microscopy of Lingzhi spores

On account of conserving natural resource, nowadays, short log or tree branches, instead of the entire tree trunk, were used for the cultivation. Nonetheless, tree-cutting for wood is still detrimental to the environment. Thus, the bag cultivation method was developed.

In the bag cultivation of Lingzhi (Fig. 3-8), polyethylene or polypropylene plastic bags are used. The medium materials may include vegetation or crop waste, such as, corn stalks, cotton seed hull, grass, wood sawdust, sugarcane pulp, wheat bran, as well as sugar, gypsum, calcium carbonate, etc. After heat sterilization of the bagged medium, Lingzhi cultivars are inoculated. In time, hyphaes appear and fruiting bodies follow in the culture bags under the required conditions on temperature, humidity and sunlight exposure.

Log cultivation is to grow Lingzhi on logs that are pre-sterilized. The mycelia appear first on the inoculated log, followed by the fruiting body under required conditions. This cultivation method is more closely related to the natural situations. The needed growth period of Lingzhi, however, tends to be longer, the fruiting body bigger, heavier and

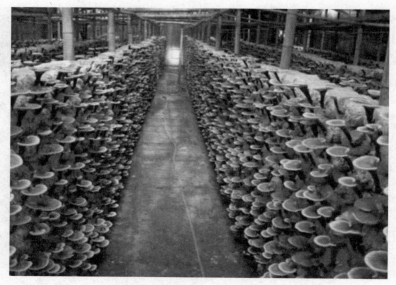

Fig. 3-8 Bag cultivated Lingzhi close to maturation.

better shaped than that of the bag cultivated counterpart.

Both log and bag cultivations require burying the logs or bags in ground after mycelia have spread. By doing so, a more stable temperature may be maintained to facilitate fruiting body development. Thus, soil and water conditions on site directly affect the final quality of Lingzhi. In particular, the heavy metals and pesticide residues are of concern, because these contaminants can be easily transferred to the fruiting body through its hyphaes.

Consequently, high quality Lingzhi products can only be obtained through the use of selected cultivars, followed by cultivation under acceptable environmental and growth conditions. Adherence to the organic agriculture practices in cultivating Lingzhi may prove to be necessary and prudent for the industry that wants to produce the products with the highest possible quality.

 Submerged fermentation for Lingzhi mycelia

The method of submerged fermentation applies a liquid medium to grow hyphaes, followed by collecting the metabolic substances and isolating the functional ingredients. Lingzhi cultivars are firstly inoculated in the liquid medium in a sealed fermentation vessel. Germ-free air is injected in the vessel with constant stirring to encourage mycelial growth under controlled temperature. By means of filtration and concentration, the metabolites of interest are collected. This engineered process has the advantages of a shortened production cycle, increased productivity, consistent product quality and lower cost. It is, therefore, becoming an emerging mass production technology for producing functional components of Lingzhi.

 Lingzhi's "genealogy" revealed by DNA fingerprinting

For a long time, fungal taxonomists classified Lingzhi according to the color, shape, and size of the macroscopic fruiting body, the appearance of the microscopic basidiospore or the composition and arrangement of the mycelium. Due to the homonyms and synonyms in existence, the traditional classification approach has proven unreliable. The more accurate method is to apply the molecular biology principle using Lingzhi's genetic characteristics to identify the species.

Chinese pharmacopoeia specifies that only the red Lingzhi (*G. lucidum*) and purple Lingzhi (*G. sinense*) can be considered medicinal materials. The National Food and Drug Administration allows *G. lucidum, G. sinense* and Songshan Lingzhi (*G. tsugae*) to be classified as health food ingredients. However, in practice, confusions continue to arise due to misunderstanding on the customary names, incorrect strain identification and/or unethical business operations. Quality of Lingzhi products on the market has been inconsistent to say the least. The result does not only affect the market and clinical applications, but also pharmacological study on Lingzhi.

Luo et al (2005) collected 30 Lingzhi specimens in China for a DNA fingerprinting analysis to determine their genetic relationships. The samples included one *G. applanatum*, one *G. capense*, 17 *G. lucidum*, one *G. japonicum*, two *G. tsugae*, one *ganoderma sp.*, one *G. formosanum*, one *G. atrum*, one *G. sinense*, one *G. shandongense* and one *G. sanmingense*. The result showed that the greatest majority of these strains were *G. lucidum* (i.e., 17 out of 30), which was followed by *G. sinense* (6 samples), *G. tsugae* (4 samples), and 3 inconclusive specimens. The report also indicated that serious confusion existed regarding the names of Lingzhi cultivars, particularly between *G·ucidum* and *G. tsugae*.

Luo, L.Z., Lin, S.Q, Xie, B.G., et al. DNA fingerprinting analysis of ganoderma lucidum strains. *Journal of Edible Fungi*, 2005, 12 (3): 7-13

 ## Organic cultivation of Lingzhi

Quality of the Lingzhi fruiting body depends on cultivars selection and control of the entire cultivation process. The guidelines stipulated in the *Good Agriculture Practice* (GAP) by the National Food and Drug Administration should be stringently adhered to. Personnel training, fungal cultivars identification and selection, medium materials, soil/water/air quality, fertilizer or pesticide applications, controls on temperature/humidity/sunlight, as well as oxygen and carbon dioxide contents can all critically and directly affect the quality of the final products.

"Organic cultivation" requires the entire farming processes to abide by specific rules and regulations set forth by either national government agencies or international certification authorities. The organic concept follows the laws of nature and ecology. It intends to protect the environment, as well as the consumers. The requirements for certi-

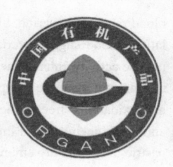

fied organic agriculture and processing could be difficult and costly to comply with. Nevertheless, the objective of the program and its guidelines are scientifically sound and ought to be followed as much as possible.

Lingzhi's active components and pharmacological effects

Lingzhi fruiting body contains sugars (including reducing sugars and polysaccharides), triterpenes, steroids, amino acids, protein, coumarin glycosides, nucleosides, alkaloids, volatile oils, resins, lipids, minerals, etc. The mycelium has similar compositions, except that its triterpene content is lower than the fruiting body. In the spores, unsaturated and saturated fatty acids, polysaccharides, nucleosides, triterpenes, etc. are found.

In the following, the pharmacological effects of the active components are briefly described.

(A) **The water extract of fruiting body and its polysaccharides/ polysaccharide peptides:**

Immune regulation, anti-tumor, protection from radiotherapy and chemotherapy-induced injuries, analgesic, sedating and cardiac anti-ischemic effects, cerebral hypoxia-reoxygenation injury avoidance,

blood pressure lowering, blood lipid regulation, blood sugar lowering, DNA polymerase activity enhancement, nucleic acid
and protein syntheses, hypoxia tolerance,
anti-oxidation, free radical scavenging,

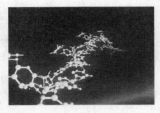

antiaging, chemical and immunological liver injury prevention, anti-
gastric ulcer, etc. are among the known functions associated with the
watersoluble components in Lingzhi fruiting body.

(B) Alcohol extract of the fruiting body and its triterpenes:

In addition to the liver-protecting,
an titumor, analgesic, sedative and anti-
oxidative effects listed above for the poly-
sac charides and/or polysaccharide peptides, the alcohol extract also showed, in
vitro, the inhibitive effects on tumor growth,

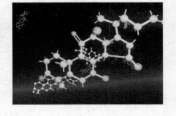

human immunodeficiency virus (HIV), histamine release, angiotensin-
converting enzyme activity, cholesterol synthesis, platelet aggregation,
etc.

(C) Spore powder extract:

It has been found to have immunity modulation, immunosup
pressive action on rat myositis, blood sugar lowering, blood lipid regulation, sedative and hypnotic effects. In vitro, it exhibited the ability
to retard tumor growth leading to eventual death of the tumor cells.
The spore oil could also lower blood lipids, prevent chemical-induced
liver damage, regulate immunity and inhibit tumor growth.

(D) Other active components:

Lingzhi-8 (LZ-8) protein was reported to have immunomodulatory
activity. The steroids showed a protective effect on cerebral hypoxia-

reoxygenation injury and anti-oxidative, free radical-scavenging activity. Adenosine in Lingzhi reduced serum aldolase in mice in experimental myotonia disease, inhibited platelet aggregation and prevented hypoxia. And, its alkaloid A and B showed anti-inflammatory characteristics in studies.

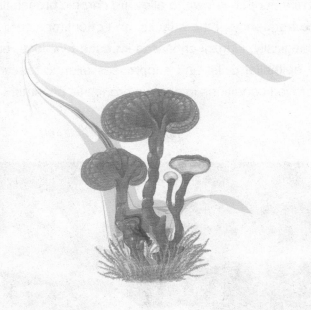

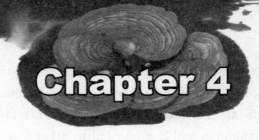

Chapter 4

Prevention and Treatment of Chronic Bronchitis with Lingzhi

Author's prompt: Through its ability to "strengthen and reinforce a person's natural defense system", according to TCM belief, Lingzhi has been known to alleviate chronic bronchitis symptoms, reduce frequency of the attacks, and oftentimes cure the disease. Physiologically, Lingzhi enhances immune functions, protects respiratory epithelial cells, and suppresses allergic reactions resulting in improved conditions in chronic bronchitis patients.

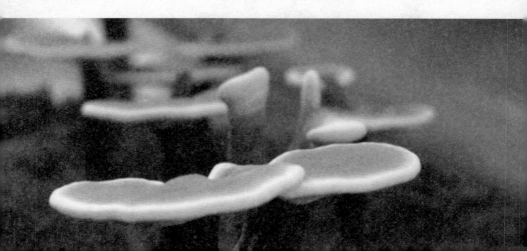

Chronic bronchitis

Chronic bronchitis is a common disease. The main symptoms include coughing
with thick white or yellow (when infection
occurs) sputum. The disease may last a long
period of time, and often recurs in winter.
Smoking, cold or flu, inhaling dust, allergies,
weather changes and air pollution are common stimulants that aggravate the bronchial
and tracheal mucus. As a result, the mucosa
thickens with increased secretion from the
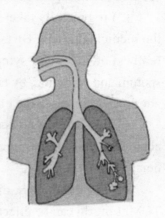
glands narrowing the respiratory passages. Partially blocked pipes pre-
vent free air passage and encourage bacterial growth. Repeated infections
on the pipes lead to permanent bronchial and tracheal mucus thickening
and cicatrization. This can further affect the lungs, such as, with chronic
obstructive lung disease (COPD). Clinically antitussive, expectorant
and anti-asthmatic drugs are used to relief the symptoms. In acute cases,
anti-infective drugs are used to control infection.

 ## Therapeutic efficacy of Lingzhi on chronic bronchitis

Since 1970s, Lingzhi has been known to be effective in treating
chronic bronchitis and asthma. As medication, Lingzhi showed the following characteristics:

(1) The clinical reports from 11 hospitals on 1,180 patients indicated
an average effective rate of 80%. The highest curing rate reached 97.6%,
while the lowest 60.0%. Significant efficacy (including clinical control
and recent cure) fluctuated between 75% and 20%. The disparity might

be related to patient's conditions, products and dosages applied and/or the treatment implemented.

(2) It generally takes 1-2 weeks after the administration to show the medicinal effect. By taking Lingzhi, significant improvements are realized on the major symptoms of chronic bronchitis, i.e., coughing, sputum and wheezing, by taking Lingzhi. Extended treatment with Lingzhi further increases the efficacy (Fig. 4-1).

(3) Lingzhi has no bactericidal effect. When infection occurs or in acute bronchitis attacks, appropriate drugs must be administered without delay (Fig. 4-2).

(4) For these cases, diagnosed as "cold and insufficiency type" by TCM, Lingzhi can be effective. In these cases, the patients are weak and have chills, coughing and excessive phlegm with white sputum. On the other hand, when the lungs and tracheae are infected, the patient coughs without sputum or spits out thick, yellowish phlegm. Lingzhi should be used only to supplement regular drugs.

(5) As a supplement, Lingzhi products considerably strengthen the body. They can improve the sleep quality, appetite, energy and resistance to cold and flu.

(6) Few side effects are known in the use of Lingzhi. In the same clinical report as shown above, there was hardly any side effects found among the 1,810 chronic bronchitis patients treated with Lingzhi. Clinical trials also showed no significant toxicity on heart, liver and kidney and other vital organs. This conclusion coincides with what TCM literature indicated: "Lingzhi is mild and non-toxic." The very rare side effects that have been reported include dizziness, dryness of nose and mouth, nose bleeding, stomach discomfort and constipation. And, these symptoms disappeared after continued treatment with Lingzhi.

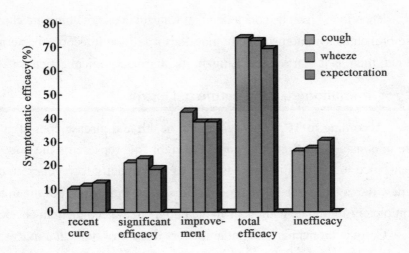

Fig.4-1 Symptomatic efficacy of Lingzhi on chronic bronchitis
The number of cases: cough: 375 cases; wheeze: 354 cases; expectoration: 367 cases

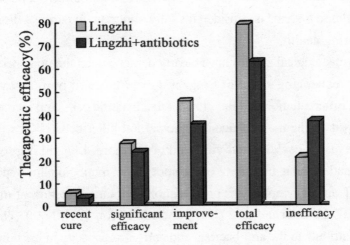

Fig.4-2 Therapeutic efficacy of Lingzhi on chronic bronchitis
Lingzhi group: 392 cases; Lingzhi plus antibiotic group: 81cases

Therefore, it can be concluded that Lingzhi does not eliminate chronic bronchitis symptoms directly, nor does it kill the infectious bacteria. What, then, is it that renders Lingzhi its pharmacological efficacy?

Immunoregulating nature of Lingzhi

According to TCM theory, human health and disease coexist and are in constant conflict. The good and right "qi" represents the body's resistance to evil or diseases, as well as the capacity to regenerate or renew damaged parts. In treatment of diseases, thus, does not mean to completely annihilate pathogens in the body, but to keep them in check.

Chronic bronchitis is an inflammatory disease of bronchial mucosa. Its complex mechanism involves bacterial infection, environmental pollution and immune dysfunction. Infection and pollution are the external factors, while dysfunctional immunity is due to inadequate "qi". Hence, treatment to upgrade "qi", or "strengthen and reinforce a person's natural defense system" is considered vitally important in curing a disease and restoring health.

Pharmacological studies have clearly demonstrated the non-specific immunity-enhancing effect of Lingzhi. For instance, it promotes proliferation, differentiation and functions of the dendritic cells, and increases phagocytosis of the macrophage and the natural killer cells(NK), which kill the invasive bacteria and viruses. Furthermore, Lingzhi improves humoral and cellular immunity by promoting immunoglobulin generation, the T and B lymphocytes proliferation, cytokine secretion of interleukin-1(IL-1), interleukin-2 (IL-2) and interferon γ (IFNγ). These can all contribute to the anti-bacteria and anti-virus capacity in the human body. Interestingly, Lingzhi is capable of restoring the immune functions when a body's immunity is suppressed by other factors (Fig. 4-3). The polysaccharides peptide in Lingzhi can protect macrophages from being damaged by the oxidant, tert-butyl hydroperoxide (tBOOH). Under an electron microscope, the villi on the surface of a marcrophage can be observed clearly. The villi practically disappear when the marcrophage is damaged by tBOOH. Yet, by adding Lingzhi polysaccharides peptide, the villi are protected (Fig. 4-3).

In addition, Lingzhi can protect ciliated columnar epithelial cells, caliciform cells and cartilaginous tissue of trachea, and relieve pathological changes of the chronic inflammation caused by smog inhalation.

It is apparent that Lingzhi's ability to treat chronic bronchitis lies in its immunity-enhancing function. By virtue of immunity improvement, cold prevention, stimulant reduction and inflammation avoidance, tracheobronchitis could be alleviated. In other words, TCM theory of "strengthening and reinforcing a person's natural defense system" is indeed the base of Lingzhi's effective treatment for chronic bronchitis.

The polysaccharides and triterpenes in Lingzhi also have an anti-allergic effect. By suppressing the allergic reaction of the skin and the release of anaphylactic mediators, the respiratory autoimmune inflamma-

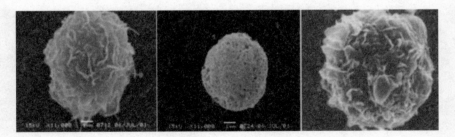

Fig4-3 Protective effect of *Ganoderma lucidum* polysaccharides peptide (GLPP) on macrophage oxidative injury induced by oxidant tBOOH. Left: macrophages in normal group; Middle: macrophages in tBOOH oxidative damage group, Right: macrophages treated with tBOOH and GLPP.

tory response induced by anaphylactogen could be prevented.It could reduce the inflammatory cells in tracheae and respiratory passages, the inflammatory mediators (such as, histamine and prostaglandin E2) and the release of eosinophil activating chemokine. Since allergy is another important factor involving the onset of chronic bronchitis or asthma, Lingzhi's application for the prevention and treatment of these diseases can be logically understood.

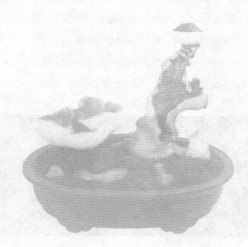

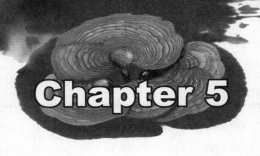

Chapter 5

Prevention and Treatment of
Hyperlipidemia with Lingzhi

Author's prompt: To administer Lingzhi alone or with lipid-lowering drugs can decrease serum cholesterol, triglycerides and low-density lipoprotein (LDL), and increase high density lipoprotein (HDL). Lingzhi can also reduce blood viscosity and improve hemorheological disorders. Its liver protection effect helps prevent or reduce injury on the liver caused by lipid-lowering drugs. With its lipid regulating function, Lingzhi is also effective for cardiovascular and cerebrovascular protection.

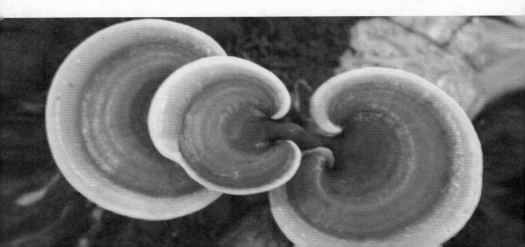

Hyperlipidemia

There are two sources for human beings to acquire lipids. One is endogenous, which is synthesized in the cells in our body. The other is exogenous, or coming from food intake. When the external source of lipids increases, body cells synthesize less, while metabolic activities and excretion increased, in order to maintain a balance, and vise versa. In the case of high lipid consumption or an inadequacy in the metabolism to reduce lipid, the balance is disturbed resulting in "hyperlipidemia" (high blood lipid syndrome). Clinically, the plasma lipids and/or lipo-protein (except high density lipoprotein, HDL) contents in blood exceed the normal levels. These conditions are believed to cause atherosclerosis, hardening of the blood vessels.

In general, tests of serum total cholesterol, triglycerides, LDL and HDL are performed for the diagnosis of hyperlipidemia. For adults after fasting, the level of the total serum cholesterol is greater than 5.72 mmol/L and that of triglyceride 1.70 mmol/L is considered a patient with hyper-lipidemia. For the marginal cases, the total cholesterol is between 5.2 and 5.7 mmol/L.

LDL can be oxidized to ox-LDL by cholesterol oxidase or supero-xide anions in the body. Superoxide anions are highly atherogenic caus-ing the blood vessel hardening. Increased LDL level risks coronary heart disease. On the other hand, HDL plays a very different role in this regard. It works against atherosclerosis by transferring excessive chole-sterol in the body to the liver to be converted to harmless substances. Thus, the more HDL, the better it is to our health. The ideal conditions are when HDL is high and LDL low.

Hyperlipidemia can be effectively treated through appropriate diet, routine physical activities and lipid-lowering drugs, such as lovastatin, simvastatin, etc.

 ## Therapeutic efficacy of Lingzhi on hyperlipidemia

Lingzhi alone or combined with other lipid-lowering drugs is effective on treating hyperlipidemia. On therapeutic applications, Lingzhi showed the following characteristics:

(1) In varying degrees, Lingzhi lowers serum cholesterol, triglyceride, β-lipoprotein and LDL, and increases HDL.

(2) It reduces blood and plasma viscosity and improve hemorheological properties of the blood facilitating blood flow and circulation.

(3) A synergistic effect exists when Lingzhi is used in combination with the conventional lipid-lowering drugs.

(4) Efficacy of Lingzhi in treating hyperlipidemia relates to the pathogenetic conditions, drug dosage and treatment time on a patient. Generally, mild and moderate hyperlipidemic patients and patients with a large dose of Lingzhi and long treatment period show better effect.

(5) The synthesized lipid-lowering drugs currently used for clinical purposes often cause liver damage. Taking Lingzhi or Lingzhi products along with the prescription drugs can prevent or mitigate the injuries.

(6) Patient's Improvements on appetite, sleep quality and energy can also result from administering Lingzhi.

 ## How does Lingzhi regulate blood lipid?

Pharmacological studies on rats with hyperlipidemia showed that Lingzhi and its polysaccharides reduced the serum cholesterol, LDL and triglyceride contents in the liver of the animals (Table 5-1). In contrast, it elevated serum HDL, significantly improved serum glutathione peroxi-

Table 5-1 Effect of ganoderma lucidum polysaccharides (GLP) on total cholesterol, triglycerides, HDL and LDL in hyperlipidemic rats

Groups	Dose (mg/kg)	Total cholesterol (mmol/L)	Triglyceride (mmol/L)	HDL (mmol/L)	LDL (mmol/L)
Control	-	1.35± 0.21	0.42± 0.23	1.22± 0.16	0.40± 0.20
Hyperlipidemic Group	-	9.13± 2.17$^\triangle$	1.19± 0.21$^\triangle$	0.72± 0.16$^\triangle$	7.17± 2.19$^\triangle$
GLP	200	5.52± 1.29**	0.83± 0.22**	0.84± 0.10*	5.14± 1.26**
GLP	400	6.23± 1.75**	0.82± 0.22**	0.86± 0.12*	5.20± 1.22**
GLP	800	5.85± 1.62**	0.80± 0.26**	0.89± 0.19*	4.23± 1.64**

$\bar{x} \pm s$; n=10; $^\triangle P < 0.01$, compared with Control; $^*P < 0.05$, $^{**}P < 0.01$, compared with Hyperlipidemic Group

dase (GSH-Px) and superoxide dismutase (SOD) activities, and reduced serum lipid peroxides (LPO) concentration. The results indicate that Lingzhi and its polysaccharides can regulate lipid metabolism and minimize lipid peroxidation in hyperlipidemic rats (Table 5-2).

Cellular molecular biology research demonstrated that Lingzhi significantly inhibited LDL oxidation reducing mononuclear cell's adhesion to vascular endothelial cells due to the presence of oxidized LDL and glycosylated albumin. Lingzhi also significantly reduced the expression of intercellular adhesion molecule-1 (ICAM-1) and vascular cell adhesion molecule-1 (VAM-1) that are induced by the oxidized LDL and glycosylated albumin. This, in turn, impacts the monocyte-endothelial cell interaction preventing atherosclerosis.

Additionally, Lingzhi triterpenoids are capable of suppressing not only cholesterol absorption by humans, but also the activity of the rate-limiting enzyme, 3-hydroxy-3-methylglutaryl-coenzyme A (HMG-

CoA) reductase A, in cholesterol synthesis. The result, obviously, is a lowered cholesterol content in our body.

Table 5-2 Effect of ganoderma lucidum polysaccharides (GLP) on serum LPO and enzyme activities of GSH-Px and SOD

Groups	Dose (mg/kg)	LPO (10^{-9}mol/L)	GSH-Px (U/ml)	SOD/(U/ml)
Control	-	5.12± 0.43	59.22± 5.16	5.02± 0.42
Hyperlipidemic Group	-	11.19± 0.61$^\triangle$	20.72± 6.16$^\triangle$	3.17± 0.79$^\triangle$
GLP	200	4.33± 0.42**	63.04± 8.19**	3.94± 1.26*
GLP	400	4.62± 0.32**	60.16± 6.12**	4.70± 1.22**
GLP	800	3.90± 0.26**	59.19± 6.19**	4.23± 0.94**

$\bar{x}$±s; n=10; $^\triangle P$ <0.01, compared with Control; $^*P$ <0.05, $^{**}P$ <0.01, compared with Hyperlipidemic Group

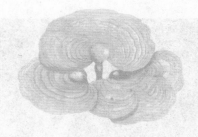

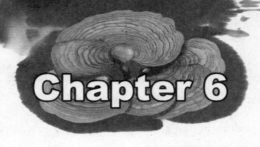

Chapter 6

Anti-Hypertensive Effects of Lingzhi

Author's prompt: Lingzhi can lower the blood pressure and improve subjective symptoms in hypertensive patients. The efficacy is particularly pronounced when it is applied in combination with conventional antihypertensive drugs. The synergy makes the control of high blood pressure easier. The treatment increases the density and diameter of the capillary blood vessels and red blood cell flow rate, while it reduces the blood viscosity resulting in improved blood circulation. Moreover, Lingzhi's effect on blood lipid regulation can directly and indirectly benefit the prevention and treatment of hypertension, as well as complications of hypertension.

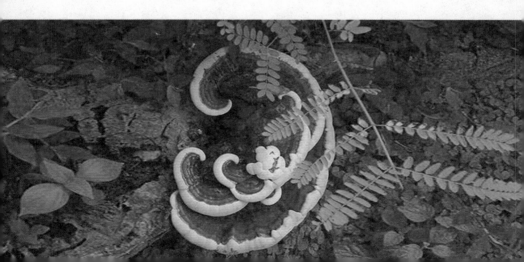

Hypertension

Hypertension is a common and frequently found cardiovascular disease (CVD) among the elderly. It may cause heart, kidney and brain complications, and is an important factor on heart attacks and strokes. The normal blood pressure for an adult is less than140/90mmHg(systolic/diastolic).

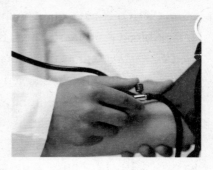

To date, the actual cause(s) of hypertension have yet been identified. Factors, such as heredity, stress, diet and obesity, have shown varying degrees of association with hypertension. Regardless, once the disease is confirmed, the patient should immediately be placed under treatment and never stop taking the drug prescribed by physician.

Clinical research conducted in China and abroad has demonstrated Lingzhi's efficacy in reducing blood pressure of and improving symptoms on hypertension patients. It is also well documented on the synergy between Lingzhi and the conventional anti-hypertension drugs.

Clinical reports on Lingzhi's efficacy for hypertension treatment

In the 1970s, physicians in China found that Lingzhi decoction and the liquid fermentation medium of the cultured Lingzhi mycelium could lower the blood pressure of and improve the symptoms on hypertension patients.

Later on, Japanese researchers, Kanmatsuse and his colleagues, reported in 1985 their experiment with 53 participating hypertension patients. The patients were divided into two groups: Group A had been diagnosed with essential hypertension according to World Health Organization (WHO) criteria, and Group B were either normal or slightly high on their blood pressure readings. Six Lingzhi tablets (i.e., 240mg freeze-dried *G. lucidum* extract/tablet) per day were administered to each person for 6 months. The results showed that the blood pressure of the patients in Group A lowered significantly. Ten percent of the patients had their systolic blood pressure decreased 20–29 mmHg and 47.5% decreased 10–19 mmHg. On the diastolic blood pressure, 17.5% of the patients decreased 10–14 mmHg and 42.5% patients decreased 5–9 mmHg. The average blood pressures were reduced from 156.6/103.5 mmHg to 136.6/92.8 mmHg with the 6 months therapy. Moreover, patients' serum total cholesterol and LDL levels were also lowered. On the other hand, no obvious changes on the blood pressures were found in Group B.

Kanmatsuse, K, et al. Studies on Ganoderma lucidum I. efficacy against hypertension and side effects. Yakugago Zasshi, 1985, 105(10):942-947

A double-blind placebo-controlled clinical study conducted by Zhang et al (1999) showed a significant synergy between Lingzhi and the conventional anti-hypertension drugs in treating patients. All 40 patients had been diagnosed with essential hypertension according to WHO criteria. The patients were given three times a day 25 mg of the angiotensin-converting enzyme inhibitor, Captopril, or 20 mg of the calcium channel blockers, Nimodipine. After no less than one month of ineffective treatment, the patients were administered a dosage of Lingzhi and the drug. The Linzhi tablets were freeze-dried extract of *G.lucidum*. Each tablet contained 55 mg *G. lucidum* extract, equivalent to 1.375 g of the fruiting body. A placebo was used that contained no

Lingzhi. Two Lingzhi or placebo tablets were given to the patients along with the prescription drug. Among 40 patients, whose average blood pressures were higher than 140/90 mmHg, 27 were given the combination therapy and 13 on placebo. In two weeks, a significant decrease on average blood pressure was observed in the group treated with Lingzhi in combination with the drug. And after three months, all patients in that group had their blood pressures dropped to 140/90 mmHg or below. Meanwhile, the aortic and capillary pressures were also decreased significantly, and the microcirculation of nail wall was considerably improved. For the patients treated with placebo, no significant changes on those indices were found. This synergetic effect between Lingzhi and anti-hypertension drugs might be the result of the improved blood circulation due to the increased density and diameter of capillary blood vessels, as well as red cell flow rate (Table 6-1, 6-2).

In addition, blood glucose levels decreased significantly from 5.81 ± 1.67 mmol/L to 4.73 ± 0.98 mmol/L ($P<0.05$) after 3 months therapy. But there were little differences in serum total cholesterol, triglycerides and HDL levels between the two groups.

In further studies, it was found that the plasma viscosity was also reduced in patients receiving the combination therapy of Lingzhi slices and the drug. The reduced blood rheological characteristics included viscosities at low and high shear rates, plasma viscosity, hematocrit values and erythrocyte sedimentation rate (Table 6-3). At the same time, the blood glucose lowered significantly and the plasma nitric oxide (NO) increased markedly in the patients administered with the combination therapy. The regression analysis showed a positive correlation between elevated NO and decreased capillary pressure. The results suggest that long-term anti-hypertension drugs combined with Lingzhi can be a solu-

Table 6-1 Changes in blood pressure (mmHg) before and after treatment

Index	Lingzhi tablet(n=27)		Placebo(n=13)	
	Pre-treatment	Post-treatment	Pre-treatment	Post-treatment
MASP	155.3± 17.5	141.2± 15.3**	161.2± 20.9	158.1± 14.3
MADP	94.4± 11.1	86.6± 7.6**	93.0± 13.1	92.9± 8.25
ASP	132.1± 16.7	120.9± 12.7**	140.2± 15.1	138.5± 15.2
ADP	78.2± 10.6	73.3± 9.5*	81.5± 14.0	83.1± 7.9
CP	51.1± 13.0	41.9± 8.8**	54.2± 10.7	55.4± 12.7

Major arteries systolic pressure (MASP); Major arteries diastolic pressure (MADP); Arterioles systolic pressure (ASP); Arterioles diastolic pressure (ADP); Capillary pressure(CP)

Values are mean± SEM; **P <0.01, *P <0.05 compared with Pre-treatment with Lingzhi tablets or Post-treatment with placebo.

Table 6-2 Changes in the microcirculation of nail wall before and after treatment

Index	Lingzhi tablet(n=27)		Placebo(n=13)	
	Pre-treatment	Post-treatment	Pre-treatment	Post-treatment
CLD(Strip/mm)	6.88± 1.26	8.28± 3.96*	7.08± 1.41	7.16± 1.85
ELD(μm)	6.76± 2.48	8.95± 2.58**	7.27± 3.33	8.88± 3.37
ALD(μm)	10.05± 3.43	12.21± 3.63**	10.85± 3.58	12.85± 5.07
RBCFR(μm/s)	444.4± 277.99	566.67± 276.22	538.46± 317.53	438.46± 258.81

Capillary loop density (CLD); Efferent limb diameter (ELD); Afferent limb diameter (ALD); Red blood cell flow rate (RBCFR)

Values are mean ± SEM; **P <0.01, *P <0.05, compared with pre-treatment with Lingzhi tablets.

tion for serious hypertension patients. Lingzhi induced serum NO increase might be one of the factors that causes the improvement in microcirculation.

Zhang, K.P. et al. Effect of Ganoderma lucidum combined with hypotensor on blood sugar, plasma NO, microcirculation and hemor-rheology in treatment refractory hypertension. J. China Microcirculation, 1999, 3(2):75-78

Therefore, Lingzhi is effective in treating hypertension, especially when it is combined with conventional anti-hypertension drugs. In addition, Lingzhi preparations could improve subjective symptoms in hypertension patients.

Table 6-3 Changes in blood rheology before and after treatment

Index	Lingzhi tablet(n=27)		Placebo(n=13)	
	Pre-treatment	Post-treatment	Pre-treatment	Post-treatment
WBVHSR(80^{-1})	5.88± 1.52	5.34± 0.72*	5.74± 1.09	5.98± 1.06
WBVLSR(20s^{-1})	7.33± 1.82	6.35± 0.96**	7.62± 1.95	7.90± 1.48
Plasma Viscosity	1.71± 0.12	1.58± 0.11**	1.74± 0.09	1.71± 0.18
Hematocrit Values(%)	0.45± 0.05	0.39± 0.04**	0.45± 0.05	0.45± 0.05
ESR(mm/h)	14.89± 12.45	10.83± 4.22*	13.62± 11.86	13.01± 9.17

Whole blood viscosity high shear rate (WBVHSR); Whole blood viscosity low shear rate (WBVLSR); Erythrocyte sedimentation rate(ESR)
Values are mean± SEM; $^{**}P<0.01$, $^*P<0.05$ compared with Pre-treatment with Lingzhi tablets or Post-treatment with placebo.

Why can Lingzhi effectively treat hypertension?

Pharmacological studies indicate that Lingzhi has anti-hypertension effect. On the spontaneously hypertension rats, feeding Lingzhi mycelium powder significantly decreased their blood pressure and cholesterol in the liver and plasma. A recent study reported that ganoderma polysaccharides lowered the superoxide in aortic vascular smooth muscles of hypertension rats to the normal level, and elevated the superoxide dismutase activity. These results suggest that the anti-oxidative and free radical-scavenging activities of Lingzhi are associated with its efficacy in treating hypertension.

At present, Lingzhi's anti-hypertension effect is believed to relate to the triterpenoids it contains. For instance, 5 triterpenoid compounds isolated from the 70% methanol extract of *G. lucidum*, i.e., ganoderic acid A, K and S, and ganoderol A and B, showed the inhibitory activity on angiotensin-converting enzyme (ACE). High ACE activity can lead to rise on blood pressure. Thus, by suppressing ACE activity, the triterpenoids can indirectly reduce symptoms of hypertension.

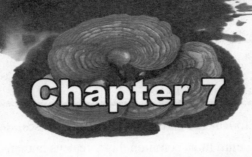

Chapter 7

Preventive and Therapeutic Effect of Lingzhi on Diabetes Mellitus

Author's prompt: Preliminary clinical trials found that Lingzhi preparation reduced the blood glucose in some patients, and enhanced the efficacy of hypoglycemic drugs. With its blood lipid-regulating and whole blood/plasma viscosity-reducing functions, Lingzhi could conceivably improve the hemorheology on patients. Thus, while the hypoglycemic drugs lower the blood sugar, Lingzhi helps delay the onset of cardiovascular and cerebrovascular diseases for the diabetic patients.

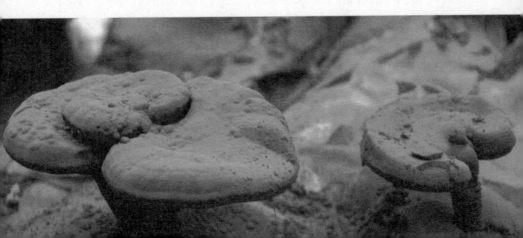

Diabetes mellitus

Next to cancers and cardiovascular diseases, diabetes mellitus has become the third most common that threatens human health. The number of diabetes cases continues to rise in China. In some metropolitan areas, the patient rate has reportedly reached beyond 10% of the population. The disease is closely related to the dietary, hereditary, environmental and immunological factors. Major clinical symptoms of diabetes include high blood glucose, excessive thirst (polydipsia), food-craving (polyphagia), frequent urination (polyuria), weight-loss (emaciation), fatigue, reduced resistance to diseases, etc. The diagnosis criterion for high blood glucose is the fasting blood glucose (FBG) at or above 140mg/dl (7.8mmol/L) or the 2-hour post-prandial blood glucose (PBG) at or above 200mg/dl (11.1mmol/L). Recently, the International Committee on the Diagnosis and Classification of Diabetes Mellitus recommended reducing FBG from 140 mg/dl to 126 mg/dl, and setting the normal level at less than 110mg/dl. Growing evidence indicates that risk of diabetes mellitus increases when FBG level reaches 100mg/dl in humans.

Diabetes per se is not a serious disease. However, it can cause a host of life threatening complications, such as (a) cardiocerebral vascular diseases, which are hypertension, coronary heart failure or cerebral ischemia resulting from high blood lipid and atherosclerosis; (b) diabetic nephropathy or renal failure induced by glomerular sclerosis; (c) diabetic retinopathy, poor vision or blindness due to retinal arteriosclerosis; and (d) multiple peripheral neuritis or gangrene of the toes. Statistically, diabetic patients died from cardio- and cerebro-vascular complications constituted more than 60% of the death, and about 12% from renal disease. Therefore, in addition to controlling the blood glucose, diabetes mellitus therapy needs also to include prevention and treatment of the associated complications. There are varieties of drugs for the blood sugar lowering purpose. They include insulin preparations and oral hypoglycemic agents, such as glibenclamide (Gilemal), glipizide (Meibida), gliclazide (Diamicron), dimethylbiguanide (Metformin), etc.

 ### Clinical reports on Lingzhi for adjuvant treatment on diabetes mellitus

At the 2002 International Symposium on *Ganoderma lucidum* in Shanghai, China, a clinical report showed that Lingzhi capsules (0.25g per capsule containing 70% of Lingzhi fruiting body extract, 20% of Lingzhi spores and 10% of a filler) significantly enhanced the efficacy of conventional oral hypoglycemic drugs on the Type 2 diabetes patients. No significant difference was found between the FBG of the 30 patients in the Drug-Only Group and those of the 100 patients in the Drug with Lingzhi+ Group before the trial. After the treatment, the FBG among the Lingzhi+Drug patients decreased significantly, and they also significantly differed from those of the Drug-Only patients. On the other hand, there were no significant changes on the fasting blood insulin (FBI) of the two groups (Table 7-1). Meanwhile, by incorporation of Lingzhi capsules in the drug treatment, a significant effect on alleviating dizziness, thirst, fatigue, body aches and weak legs was observed among the patients.

Zhang, C.Y. and Li, Y.M. Clinical investigation of Green Valley Lingzhi capsule on Type 2 diabetes mellitus. In "*Ganoderma*: Genetics, Chemistry, Pharmacology and Therapeutics" Z.B. Lin ed. Beijing Medical University Press, Beijing, 2002:194-198

Another study evaluated the efficacy of Ganopoly (polysaccharides extracted from Lingzhi) in 71 Type 2 diabetes mellitus patients. These 18-year-old or older patients with normal electrocardiogram were diagnosed with the disease longer than 3 months and have never received insulin for treatment. Those who were never treated with sulfonylurea had a fasting plasma glucose (FPG) ranging from 8.9 to 16.7 mmol/L, and those sulfonylurea-treated patients had an FPG of 10 mmol/L prior to stopping the drug treatment. All participating patients were randomly divided into Treatment and Control Groups. The patients were given orally 1,800 mg Ganopoly, or a placebo, 3 times daily for 12 weeks. After fasting, glycosylated hemoglobin (HbA1c), plasma glucose, insulin and C-peptide were determined for the patients before and after a meal. The results showed that Ganopoly significantly decreased the average HbA1c in the patients, from 8.4 before the treatment to 7.6% at the end of the 12th week. Significant changes on FPG and post-prandial plasma glucose (PPG) paralleled those on HbA1c, decreasing from 13.6 to 11.8 mmol/L. In contrast, there were either no changes or slight increases in patients in the Control group who received placebo. The insulin and

Table 7-1 Effect of co-administration of Lingzhi capsules and conventional oral hypoglycemic agents on FBG and FBI levels in diabetes mellitus patients

Group	n		FBG (mmol/L)	FBI (U/ml)
Control	30	Before treatment	9.74± 1.84	9.00± 1.98
		After treatment	7.18± 2.30**	8.71± 1.65
Treatment	100	Before treatment	9.37± 1.02	8.77± 2.72
		After treatment	6.24± 1.18***△	8.43± 2.26

$\bar{x}\pm s$; **$P<0.01$, ***$P<0.001$ vs. before treatment; △$P<0.05$ vs. control

C-peptide levels of the patients at fasting or 2 hours after a meal, also showed significant differences between the two groups. All patients appeared to have no apparent side effects in taking Ganopoly during the course of the trial. The study concluded that Ganopoly could be effectively applied for treating Type II diabetes mellitus patients. Gao, Y., Lan, J., Dai, X., Ye, J. and Zhou, S. A phase I/II study of lingzhi mushroom *Ganoderma lucidum* (W.Curt.:Fr.) Lloyd (*Aphyllophoromycetideae*) extract in patients with Type II diabetes mellitus. *Int J Med Mush.* 2004, 6:33-9.

Mechanism of adjuvant therapeutic effect of Lingzhi on diabetes mellitus

As early as 1970s and1980s, pharmacological research had already recognized the hypoglycemic effect of Lingzhi. The water extract of Lingzhi fruiting bodies, when fed to mice or rat, significantly decreased their blood glucose. It was also known that the active hypoglycemic components were the *G. lucidum* polysaccharides (*Gl*-PS). Alloxan injection in a mouse can destroy the islet cells inducing high blood glucose syndrome in the animal, which is similar to the Type 1 diabetes in human. *Gl*-PS, introduced either by feeding or injection, increased the insulin level, and decreased the blood glucose in the mice injected with alloxan. Further study found that this effect of *Gl*-PS also relates to the inhibition of alloxan-induced oxygen free radical production and lipid peroxidation, as well as the protection of pancreatic islet B cells that maintains a normal function of insulin secretion. *Gl*-PS could also significantly increase the activities of hepatic glucokinase, phosphofructokinase and glucose-6-phosphate dehydrogenase, as well as decrease liver glycogen content. These findings suggest that *G. lucidum* polysaccharide's hypoglycemic effect might result from the increases in the body's antioxidation activity, serum insulin secretion, glucose metabolism and the liver and peripheral glucose utilization, as well as the protection of pancreatic islet B cells.

Gl-PS was found to play a significant role in preventing the streptozotocin-induced diabetic kidney disease in mice. It significantly reduced the pathologic change of glomerulus, as well as the protein content in urine (Fig. 7-1, 7-2). In addition, this effect was attributed to the anti-oxidation and free radical scavenging ability of the polysaccharides (Fig. 7-3). It is further understood that this anti-oxidation activity inhibited LDL oxidation and the oxidized LDL and advanced glycation end product (AGE) induced-expression of vascular endothelial cell adhesion molecule, such as intercellular adhesion molecule-1 (ICAM-1) and vascular cell adhesion molecule-1 (VCAM-1). Thereby, the mononuclear cell adhesion to vascular endothelium was restricted, and the vascular disease in diabetic patients with high blood glucose and blood lipid could be minimized or delayed.

He, C.Y., Li, W.D., Guo, S.X. et al. Effect of polysaccharides from *Ganoderma lucidum* on streptozotocin-induced diabetic nephropathy in mice.

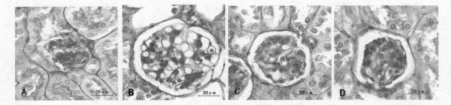

Figure 7-1 Effect of *Gl*-PS on streptozotocin-induced glomerular pathological change in diabetic kidney diseased mice
A: Control group; B: Streptozotocin-induced diabetic kidney diseased group; C: *Gl*-PS 125 mg/kg therapeutic group; D: *Gl*-PS 250 mg/kg therapeutic group

Journal of Asian Natural Products Research, 2005, 8(8):705-711.

Based on current understanding, diabetes mellitus is an autoimmune disease. Viral infection or toxic chemicals could directly or indirectly induce the immune-pathological response leading to the autoimmune islet inflammation and/or destruction of pancreatic islet cells that results in diabetes mellitus. Consequently, correcting immune abnormality has become an important element in treating diabetes. Lingzhi's immune regulating activity might, therefore, relate to its efficacy in preventing and treating diabetes mellitus. In our recent study, LPS was found to protect the mice from the immune diabetes mellitus induced by the strep-tozocin multiple low-dose (MLD-STZ) injections. The polysaccharides could not only significantly decrease blood glucose and the rate of MLD-STZ induced autoimmune diabetes in mice, but also promote the protein

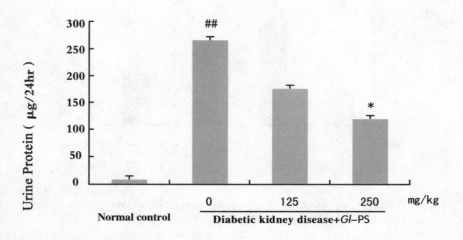

Figure 7-2 Effect of *Gl*-PS on protein content in urine of diabetic kidney diseased mice
[##] $P < 0.01$ *vs.* control, [*] $P < 0.05$ *vs.* diabetic kidney diseased group

expression of glucose transporter-2 (GLUT-2) and improve the insulin secretary function of pancreatic islet cells. In addition, by virtue of immunity improvement, Lingzhi could aid in warding off bacterial and viral infections that often take place on diabetic patients.

At present, therapies for diabetes mellitus almost always include measures to prevent and/or treat the complications, besides using insulin

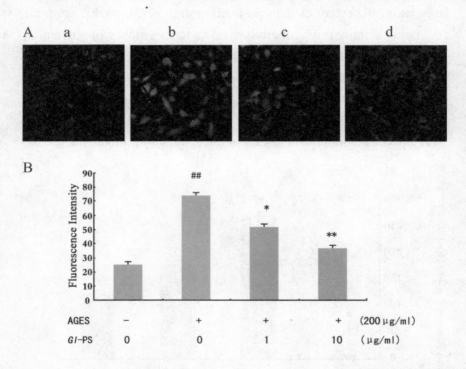

Figure 7-3 Inhibitive effect of *Gl*-PS on the generation of oxygen free radicals induced by AGE in vascular endothelium cells
A: Red fluorescence pictures showing oxygen free radicals in vascular endothelium cells - the brighter the red color, the more free radicals generated.
a: Control; b: AGE Control; c&d: AGE+*Gl*-PS
B: Digitized fluorescent intensities as converted from a-d in A
$P<0.01$ *vs.* control; * $P<0.05$, ** $P<0.01$ *vs.* AGE

and oral hypoglycemic agents to control blood glucose. Although Lingzhi can decrease the blood glucose, continuing hypoglycemic drug administration is necessary for most patients. When blood glucose is under control and maintained at normal and stable level, supplementing the drug treatment with Lingzhi may allow dose reduction to minimize adverse reactions from the drugs. Regardless, Lingzhi's hepatic protective effect should be beneficial in reducing or preventing potential liver damage by hypoglycemic drugs.

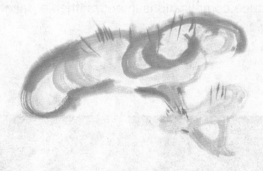

Chapter 8

Prevention and Treatment with Lingzhi for Neurasthenia

Author's prompt: Lingzhi per se are not sedative hypnotics. It is by way of recovering the dysfunctional nerve-endocrine-immune system and blocking the vicious cycle of long-term insomnia can Lingzhi improve sleep, uplift the spirit, rejuvenate memory, energize body and reduce complications in neurasthenia patients.

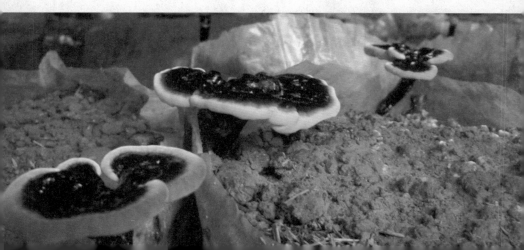

Neurasthenia

Neurasthenia is a common disease in modern society. Sleep disorder is the primary symptom, which includes difficulty in falling asleep and/or inability to sleep sound and solid for a reasonable period of time. A survey among the middle-aged Chinese in various provinces revealed that 66% of the adults had insomnia, dreamed too much or were having difficulty falling asleep, and 57% of the population had memory impairment.

Long-term neurasthenia and insomnia could lead to central nervous system disorder, neuron excitability or inhibition dysfunction, resulting in the autonomic nerve (sympathetic nerve and parasympathetic nerve) function disorder syndrome. Symptoms of the disease may include headaches, dizziness, failing memory, loss of appetite, palpitation, short breath, etc. As the disease progresses, dysfunctions in the endocrine and immune systems may be diagnosed. Impotence, irregular menstruation or immunity deficiency could result. Eventually, the disordered nerve-endocrine-immune system becomes a part of a vicious cycle, which further deteriorates the neurasthenia patient's health and well-being. Common hypnotics can only treat the neurasthenia symptoms. They do not resolve the root problem that lies in the nerve-endocrine-immune system of the patient.

 Rejuvenation of nerve-endocrine-immune system with Lingzhi

Lingzhi has a significant effect on insomnia for the neurasthenia patients. Within 1–2 weeks after the administration, patient's sleep quality, appetite, weight-gain, memory and energy improved, and palpitation, headache and complications are relieved or eliminated. Actual therapeutic effect depends on dosage and treatment period of the specific cases. In general, larger doses and longer treatment periods tend to yield better results. For those patients diagnosed by TCM practice as "deficient in qi (vital energy) and blood or the heart and spleen" (shown with the symptoms, such as palpitation, forgetfulness, insomnia, loss of appetite, abdominal distension, loose bowel, sallow face, weak pulse), Lingzhi's efficacy may be more pronounced than in other types of patients.

For chronic bronchitis, coronary heart disease, hepatitis or hypertension patients, who also suffer from insomnia, Lingzhi can not only help improve their sleep quality but also aid in the treatment for their main diseases. Pharmacological study showed that Lingzhi significantly decreased the autonomic activities, shortened the sleep latency induced by pentobarbital, and increase the sleep time on pentobarbital-treated mice, indicating that Lingzhi had a sedation effect on the test animals.

Aside from its sedative function, Lingzhi's homeostasis regulation effect might also have contributed to its efficacy on neurasthenia and insomnia. Through homeostasis regulation, Lingzhi could revive the disordered nerve-endocrine-immune system interrupting the neurasthenia-insomnia vicious cycle. Thereby, patient's sleep could be improved and other symptoms relieved or eliminated.

These effects of Lingzhi for neurasthenia and insomnia appear in agreement with the "soothing the nerves," "promoting intelligence" and "forgetting-not" characteristics of Lingzhi as described in *Shennong Material Medica*.

 Clinical reports on neurasthenia treatment with Lingzhi

In the 1970s, the Integrated Traditional and Western Medicine Group at the Department of Psychiatry, Third Affiliated Hospital, Beijing Medical College in Beijing, found that Lingzhi had a significant effect on neurasthenia as well as residue neurasthenic syndrome at the schizophrenia recover stage (NS). In 100 of the clinical cases, 50 had been diagnosed with neurasthenia, and 50 with NS. Tablets containing 0.25g Lingzhi powder made from the *Ganoderma lucidum* fermentation liquid were used for the treatment. The patients were given 4 tablets each time, 3 times a day, for oral administration. Some of these patients took 4-5 tablets each time, twice a day. The treatment lasted more than one month, 6 months being the longest. The therapeutic effect was evaluated, and classified into 3 categories: (a) "significantly improved" cases with disappearance of major symptoms; (b) "improved" cases with partial disappearance of major symptoms; and (c) "not affected" cases with no change observed after one-month treatment. The results indicated that, after more than a month of the treatment, 61 cases improved significantly, 35 cases improved and 4 cases were not affected. Thus, the total effective rate was 96%. The rate of significantly improved cases for neurasthenia, 70%, were greater than NS (i.e., 52%). The efficacy on patients with "deficiency in qi and blood" was better than their counterparts. Nonetheless, the symptoms significantly improved in both neurasthenia and NS patient groups after the treatment (Table 8-1). Most patients began to show improvements in 2-4 weeks of treatment. The significantly improved cases increased during the first 2-4 months. After 4 months, the treatment did not produce further improvement, however.

Few side effects from the administration of the Lingzhi tablets were found. Among those reported, 8 were constipation, 7 dry mouth and bitter taste, 3 dry pharynx and blistering in mouth, 3 lack of appetite, 3 abdominal distension or diarrhea, 2 acid stomach reflux and 1 stomachache. These side effects disappeared in the course of continuous treatment.

In recent years, more clinical trials with placebo, or positive drug control, were conducted. They have further confirmed Lingzhi's efficacy on neurasthenia and insomnia.

Table 8-1 Efficacy of Lingzhi tablet on neurasthenia and NS

Symptoms	Neurasthenia		NS	
	Total cases	Effective cases	Total cases	Effective cases
Insomnia	45	40	40	32
Lack of appetite	30	27	26	20
Body weakness	27	21	31	24
Low energy/poor memory	17	13	18	16
Headache, dizziness	16	8	7	3
Upset/mental instability	10	4	11	8
Flustered, short breath	7	5	4	1
Dyspepsia, loose stool	6	4	2	1
Lethargy	2	2	1	1
Impotency, spermatorrhea	2	2		
Menstrual disorder	3	3		
Tinnitus	3	3		
Sensitivity to coldness	5	2	1	1
Compulsive symptom	1	1	2	
Frequent dreams	11	3	3	3
Waist aches	1	1		

Based on China's classification and diagnose criteria for mental disorders (CCMD-2-R), Wang, et al (2001) selected 120 insomnia patients with "deficiencies in the heart and spleen". The subjects aged between 18 and 65, and had their Pittsburgh Sleep Quality Index (PSQI) greater than 7 (the greater the score the poorer the patient's sleeping quality is). The trial was a double blind, parallel controlled, random experiment. The Treatment and Control Group each had 60 participants. There were no significant differences on sex, age, length and severity of the disease or PSQI between the two groups. The patients in the Treatment Group were orally administered 40 ml of Lingzhi mycelium liquid each time, 3 times a day. The Control Group took 4 Lingzhi mycelium tablets each time, 3 times daily. The trial lasted 4 weeks. No sedative drugs were allowed during the trial. PSQI, sleep, awake time and mental state after wakening, as well as heartbeat and blood pressure of the patients were recorded before and after the treatments. The therapeutic effects on insomnia and TCM diagnosis of the symptoms were determined according to the *Instruction for Clinical Research Using the New Traditional Chinese Medicine Principles*. Patient's sleep quality was evaluated according to the PSQI scores. The decreasing rate of PSQI was calculated according to the following formula: PSQI decreasing rate=(score before treatment — score after treatment)/(score after treatment)×100%. When the decreasing rate was 76%–100%, it was considered as "clinical control;" at the rate of 51%–75%, "significant efficacy;" at the rate of 25%–50%, "efficacy;" and, at the rate of less than 25%, "inefficacy."

The results obtained from the trial were:

(1) On insomnia, 15 patients belonged to clinical controls, 24 had the significant efficacy rating (i.e., 65% control plus significant rating),

18 the efficacy rating (i.e., 95% total effective rating) and 3 the inefficacy rating in the Treatment Group. In the Control Group, 7 were clinical
controls, 19 had the significant efficacy rating (i.e., 43.3% control plus
significant ratings), 26 the efficacy rating (i.e., 86.7% total effective
rating), and 8 the inefficacy rating. The Treatment Group had a better
result than the Control Group.

(2) On sleep quality, 10 patients were clinical controls, 19 had the
significant efficacy rating (i.e., 48.3% control plus significant ratings),
27 the efficacy rating (i.e., 93.3% total effective rating), and 3 the inefficacy rating in the Treatment Group. In the Control Group, 3 were clinical
controls, 20 had the significant efficacy rating (i.e., 38.3% control plus
significant ratings), 25 the efficacy rating (i.e., 80% total effective rating),
and 2 the inefficacy rating. The Treatment Group showed a better efficacy than the Control Group.

(3) On the symptom relief defined by TCM, 10 were clinical controls, 27 had the significant efficacy rating (i.e., 61.7% control plus significant ratings), 21 the efficacy rating (i.e., 96.7% total effective rating),
and 2 the inefficacy rating in the Treatment Group. In the Control Group,
5 were clinical controls, 17 had the significant efficacy rating (i.e., 36.7%
control plus significant ratings), 27 the efficacy rating (i.e., 81.7% total
effective rating), and 11 the inefficacy rating. The Treatment Group was
also better than the Control Group. The symptoms relieved were excep-
tional for both groups with respect to insomnia, frequent dreams, palpitation, forgetfulness, bodily exhaustion, lack of appetite, abdominal distension after eating, sallow face, loose stool, pale tongue with teeth marks,
thin lingual, weak pulse, etc. On palpitation and pale face, the Treatment
Group showed a superior effect than the Control Group.

(4) On the effects after 4 weeks treatment, either individual or group

PSQI scores for the two groups showed significant differences before and after the treatment. The Treatment Group was better than the Control Group in regard to sleep quality and daytime functions. No adverse reactions due to the treatments were observed on all patients. The results indicated that both Lingzhi mycelium liquid and Lingzhi tablets were effective in treating insomnia patients diagnosed with "deficiencies in the heart and spleen". The mycelium liquid appeared better in efficacy than the tablets. It was attributed to the larger dosage applied and greater bio-availability of the mycelium liquid.

Wang, X.L., Men, Z.Y.and Wang, C.P. Treatment of *Ganoderma lucidum* mycelium liquid on 60 cases of insomnia. Journal of China Medicine, 2001, 16(1):47-49

Zhou et al (2004) studied the effects of a Lingzhi preparation on insomnia using a parallel, open-controlled, random clinical trial based on the requirements stipulated for research on the protected Chinese medicinal materials. One hundred insomnia in-patients and those who could follow instructions well were selected for the trial. They were all diagnosed with "deficiencies in the heart and spleen" by TCM practice. A treatment and a control group of 50 patients each were formed with no significant differences on age and pre-treatment scores. Other than one patient in the Control Group dropped out, all participants followed through the entire trial. The diagnosis criteria used by the western medicine included: (1) the typical insomnia symptoms of difficulty in falling asleep or returning to sleep, light sleep, frequent wakening; early morning wake-up, failure to fall asleep at night, less than 5 hours sleep per day and daytime drowsiness; and (2) a history of recurrence. The diagnosis criteria employed by TCM were: deficiencies in the heart and spleen with symptoms of insomnia, exhaustion, weakness, palpitation, fluster, forgetfulness, loss of taste, abdominal distension after eating, loose stool, light tongue and weak pulse.

TCM divided the severity of the symptoms into 3 levels: slight (scored 1), moderate (scored 2) and server (scored 3). In a 4-week trial, the patients in the Treatment Group (including an open test group) took 2 g of Lingzhi instant granules, 3 times a day, while those in the Control Group had 8-9 Guipi pills (a Chinese patented medicine for invigorating the spleen and nourishing the heart), 3 times daily. The criteria for evaluating the degree of cure were:

(1) Based on TCM, (a) "clinical recovery," i.e., disappearance of clinical symptoms with a severity score of 0; (b) "efficacy," i.e., disappearance of most of the clinical symptoms with 90% reduction on the severity score; (c) "improvement," i.e., partial disappearance of clinical symptoms with 70% reduction on the severity score; and, (d) "ineffective," i.e., either no improvement or worsening with less than 30% reduction on the severity score.

(2) Based on the insomnia symptoms, (a) "clinical recovery," i.e., sleep time returned to normal or more than 6 hours, slept deeply and became energetic after up waking-up; (b) "efficacy," i.e., sleep was significantly improved, sleep time increased by more than 3 hours, and slept relatively deeply; (c) "improvement," i.e., symptoms were relieved with sleep time increased by less than 3 hours; (d) "ineffective," i.e., insomnia was not improved or became worse.

The results are shown in number and percentage (in parentheses) of the clinical recovery, effect, improved and ineffective ratings, as 16 (32%), 16 (32%), 14 (28%) and 4 (8%), respectively, for the Treatment Group; and for the Control Group, 10 (20.41%), 13 (26.53%), 15 (30.61%) and 11 (22.45%), respectively. The total effective rate was 92% for the

Treatment Group, and 77.5% for the Control Group. There was a significant difference between the two groups (P<0.01). The changes of accumulated scores before and after treatment in the Treatment and the Control Group are shown in Table 8-2.

The results indicated that Lingzhi instant granule was effective on neurasthenia insomnia patients with the "deficiencies in the heart and spleen", and it was better than Guipi pill. There was no toxicity or adverse reaction found. The authors suggested that the therapeutic effect of Lingzhi might be due to the improved hemopenia and hematopoiesis on the patients. In addition, the sedation effect of Lingzhi might have contri-

Table 8-2 Changes on accumulated scores before and after treatment

Symptoms	Treatment group$^\triangle$			Control group		
	n	Before	After	n	Before	After
Insomnia	50	3.44± 1.15	1.2± 1.14[**]	49	2.94± 1.01	1.4± 1.19[**]
Fatigue	50	1.8± 0.57	0.48± 0.65[**]	49	1.73± 0.49	0.71± 0.65[**]
Lack of appetite	43	1.65± 0.65	0.37± 0.54[**]	47	1.53± 0.58	0.47± 0.55[**]
Palpitation	37	1.43± 0.50	0.27± 0.51[**]	34	1.53± 0.56	0.50± 0.56[**]
Abdominal distension	37	1.35± 0.48	0.27± 0.45[**]	31	1.48± 0.51	0.61± 0.62[**]
Forgetfulness	44	1.52± 0.59	0.89± 0.44[**]	41	1.51± 0.55	0.88± 0.6[**]
Loose stool	29	1.24± 0.58	0.17± 0.38[**]	25	1.48± 0.59	0.52± 0.51[**]
Total score	50	10.8± 2.96	3.26± 2.07[**]	49	10.2± 2.96	4.37± 2.21[**]

$^\triangle P$ <0.05, Comparison between Treatment and Control Group after treatment;
[**]P <0.01 Comparison between before and after treatment in a same group.

buted to its superior performance, as compared to Guipi pill.

Zhou, F.G.,Xu, H. and Ye, Y.L. Clinical observation of Lingzhi particles treated 100 cases of insomnia. Chinese Medical Science & Technology, 2004, 11(5): 309-311.

In a recent clinical report, Lingzhi syrup also showed a significant effect in treating neurasthenia of the "deficiencies in the heart and spleen" type. In that study, 240 patients were randomly divided into two groups by 2:1 ratio, i.e., 160 subjects in the Treatment Group and 80 in the Control Group. The patients in the Treatment Group were given 20 ml of the Lingzhi syrup for oral administration, 3 times a day. The Control Group took 9 g of Guipi Yanxin pills (a Chinese patented medicine similar to Guipi pill), twice daily. No other medicinal treatment for the ailment was allowed during the trial. After one month of treatment, the results showed that Lingzhi syrup yielded a total effective rate of 89.4%, while Guipi Yanxin pill, 80.0%. There was no significant difference between the two treatments. Lingzhi syrup improved the major symptoms of neurasthenia of "deficiency in the heart and spleen" type, especially insomnia, palpitation, depression, anxiety, lack of appetite, etc. This indicates Lingzhi's efficacy in tranquilizing, nourishing the heart and strengthening the spleen and stomach. No adverse reactions were observed in any of the participating patients. Neither were abnormalities detected in blood, urine, stool or hepatic and renal functions after the treatment. Thus, it was concluded that Lingzhi syrup appeared to be safe for clinical applications.

Wang, Z.Y., Liu, T.S., Zuo, Z.W. et al. Lingzhi syrup treated 160 cases of neurasthenia with deficiency of both the heart and spleen. Hunan Journal of Traditional Chinese Medicine, 2007, 23(2):54-55.

Clinical reports on memory improvement by Lingzhi

In *Shennong Material Medica*, Lingzhi was said to have the function of "promoting brain power" and "improving memory". This effect of Lingzhi was scientifically examined and confirmed by Hu (2003). The study recruited healthy, 30- to 60-year-old, high school graduates, who had not previously participated in any similar test, nor had taken drugs or health food to promote memory in a year prior to the trial. During the test, 60 participants were ranked by their memory quotient (MQ). They were randomly assigned, 30 each, to a test and a control group of subjects with equally distributed MQ.

The Test Group was given sample No. 1, which was a Lingzhi extract, 0.8 g to 1.6 g each time, twice a day. The Control Group had sample No. 2, a placebo containing starch and caramel. The participating subjects did not know whether they were taking Lingzhi extract or the placebo. After 30 days of trial, the two groups were examined again. Memorization ability of the subjects, in terms of the clinical memory scale, was evaluated using the method of the *Evaluation Procedures and Testing Methods of Functional Food* established by the Ministry of Health, China. Evaluation characteristics included the pointing memory (PM), associational learning (AL), picture free recall (PFR), nonsense figure recognition (NFR) and portrait feature association recall (PFAR). To avoid differentiations in the degree of difficulty, one half of the subjects were first given series A questions, then series B questions; and the second half in a reverse order. A same examiner tested the same subjects on a different set of questions. During the second examination, the examiners were not given a list of the group to be tested to minimize potential errors due to personal bias and/or biological rhythm of the subjects.

The raw data were converted to scaled scores for comparison and analysis. Compounded results of the scaled scores for each group were calculated, and the MQs were compared between the two groups. Both inter-and intra-group comparisons were statistically analyzed. The results are listed in Table 8-3. It showed Lingzhi's significant enhancement effects on AL, NFR, and PFAR, as well as MQ.

Table 8-3 Comparison of scaled scores and MQs of subjects in Test and Control Groups before and after treatment (x̄±s, n=30)

Tested Items	Test Group		Control Group	
	Before Treatment	After Treatment	Before Treatment	After Treatment
PM	11.83± 3.41	12.47± 1.91	11.66± 2.97	11.57± 2.28
AL	8.60± 2.24	10.73± 1.91**#	8.97± 2.34	9.43± 2.06
PFR	11.97± 3.24	11.73± 2.07	12.43± 4.29	11.73± 3.31
NFR	9.80± 1.55	11.20± 1.71**	10.93± 1.72	10.93± 1.72
PFAR	8.67± 2.37	9.97± 1.87*	9.63± 2.40	10.23± 1.91
MQ	50.83± 6.20	56.13± 4.8**##	53.67± 7.78	53.00± 7.78

Remarks: Intra-group comparison between before and after treatment, *$P<0.05$,
**$P<0.01$; group comparison between Test and Control groups, #$P<0.05$, ##$P<0.01$.

Hu, G.C. Observation on memory improving effect of Lingzhi. Zhejiang Journal of Traditional Chinese Medicine, 2003(8):362-362.

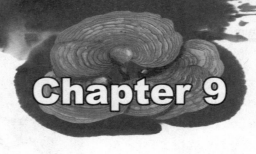

Chapter 9

Prevention and Treatment of Hepatitis with Lingzhi

Author's prompt: As a hepatoprotective drug, Lingzhi exhibits an apparent effect in protecting the liver. It has been applied for curing viral hepatitis, chemical liver injuries caused by alcohol or drugs. Lingzhi's immunoregulatory characteristic also benefits the correction of immune functional disorder of viral hepatitis. Triterpenoids in Lingzhi are believed to be the active ingredient for protecting the liver.

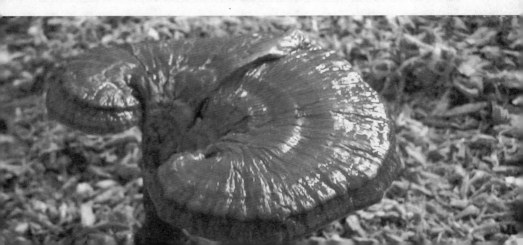

There are two kinds of hepatitis, i.e., viral and non-viral. Viral
hepatitis can be caused by different
viruses, and are classified Type A,
B, C, D and E. Type A and E are
acute, while B, C and D mostly

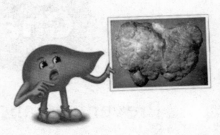

chronic. Chronic hepatitis could develop into hepatic cirrhosis or cancer.
On the other hand, non-viral hepatitis results from alcoholic and/or
chemical poisoning.

Treatment for viral hepatitis includes anti-viral, immunity regulatory
and hepatoprotective measures. Although anti-virus drugs, such as interferon, interferon inducers and lamivudine (LAM) are available at present,
these drugs are not as effective as they could be, and they have many
adverse side effects. Since immunological disturbance and hepatic injury
occur simultaneously with the viral attack in the viral hepatitis, means
to protect the liver and improve a patient's immunity cannot be overem-
phasized. Especially, when non-virus hepatitis is concerned, liver protection and immunotherapy must be implemented for an effective cure.

Therapeutic efficacy of Lingzhi on hepatitis

Though Lingzhi has no direct anti-hepatic virus effect, its immuno-
regulation and liver protection characteristics aid in treatment for viral
hepatitis along with the drugs.

In the 1970s, China began to use Lingzhi for treatment of viral hepatitis. A comprehensive clinical report indicated that the total effective
rate ranged from 73.1% to 97.0%. The best curing rate including the
clinical curing rate was 44.0%–76.5%. Indication of a cure included: (a)
reduction or disappearance of the subjective symptoms, such as fatigue,

lack of appetite, abdominal distension and pain in hepatic area; (b) normalization or lowering of the liver function tests, such as serum alanine aminotransferase (ALT); and (c) disappearance or reduction of liver and/or spleen swelling. In general, the therapeutic effect of Lingzhi is more pronounced in acute hepatitis than in chronic or persistent hepatitis. Clinically, administration of Lingzhi can prevent or reduce drug-induced liver damage. Lingzhi's liver-protective effect is expressed as "support qi of the liver and the spleen " by TCM.

Clinical reports on Lingzhi's efficacy for hepatitis treatment

Beginning in the 1970s, application of Lingzhi for hepatitis treatment continue to date. Based on the diagnostic criteria of the National Symposium on Viral Hepatitis, Hu (2001) studied the therapeutic efficacy of Lingzhi capsules on 86 chronic hepatitis B patients. In the study, except diammonium glycyrrhizinate, cape jasmine preparation, hepatocyte growth factor (HGF) and glucuronic acid lactone, no antiviral or immunoregulating drugs were given to the patients. For the duration of 1 to 2 months, the 86 patients were administered 2 Lingzhi capsules (containing 1.5 g natural Lingzhi per capsule) 3 times a day. At the same time, the control group of 50 took a packet of Xiaochaihutang granules, 3 times a day. The efficacy was evaluated according to the following indicators: clinical observations, determinations of ALT, serum bilirubin (SB), hepatitis B surface antigen (HBsAg), as well as hepatitis B virus core antigen (HBeAg) and antibody (anti-HBc). The results showed that the appetite improvement was 81 out of 86 cases (i.e., 94.2%), fatigue alleviation 80 out of 86 cases (i.e., 93.0%), abdominal distension disappearance 48 out of 52 cases (i.e., 92.3%), hepatomegaly reduction 22 out of 48 cases (i.e., 45.8%), and splenomegaly reduction 12 out of 28 cases (i.e., 42.9%) in the treatment group; and for the control group they were 39 out of 50 (i.e., 78.0%), 40 out of 50 cases (i.e., 80.0%), 28 out of 40 (i.e., 70.0%), 8 out of 33 (i.e., 24.2%) and 5 out of 19 (i.e., 26.3%), respectively. There were significant differences between the two groups. As shown in Tables 9-1 and 9-2, the rate of liver function (i.e., ALT and SB) returning to normal and the negative conversion rates of HbsAg, HbeAg and anti-HBc were considerably higher in the Treatment Group than the Control Group. It was thus concluded that Lingzhi capsules were effective in adjunctive therapy in treating chronic hepatitis B.

Table 9-1 Recovery of liver function with administration of Lingzhi capsules

Groups	ALT			SB		
	Cases Tested	Cases of Recovery	Rate%	Cases Tested	Cases of Recovery	Rate%
Lingzhi	86	82	95.3	72	66	91.7
Control	50	36	72.0	40	26	72.5

$P < 0.05$, treatment group compared with control group.

Table 9-2 Negative conversion rates of hepatitis B virus markers with Lingzhi treatment

Groups	HBsAg			HBeAg			抗-HBe		
	Cases Tested	Negative Conversion	Rate %	Cases Tested	Negative Conversion	Rate %	Cases Teste	Negative Conversion	Rate %
Lingzhi	86	14	16.3	74	38	51.4	86	13	15.1
Control	50	4	8.0	36	7	19.4	50	4	8.0

$P < 0.05$, treatment group compared with control group.

Hu, J. Analysis of 86 cases in *Ganoderma lucidum* capsule's treatment with chronic hepatitis B. Occupation and Health, 2003, 19(3): 103-104

Zhong et al (2006) compared the therapeutic effects of anti-viral drug, LAM, and LAM in combination with Lingzhi on chronic hepatitis B. The tested patients met the diagnostic criteria of viral hepatitis prevention and treatment programs established by the Chinese Medical Association at the 10th National Symposium on Viral Hepatitis and Liver Disease on September 2000. The criteria are consistent in regards to HbeAg, positive hepatitis B virus-related DNA polymerase (HBV DNA), 2 to 3 times higher than the upper limit of normal ALT, and more than 3 times upper limit of normal total bilirubin (TBil). Cases excluded for consideration were (a) infection with other hepatitis viruses (e.g., HAV, HCV, HEV, HDV and HGV), (b) diagnosis of autoimmune liver disease, (c) having fatty liver, and/or (d) with complications of diabetes or the like. Randomly divided equally among the 126 patients into two groups of treatment with LAM and LAM in combination with Lingzhi. There were no significant differences on age, sex, length of illness, using liver protective drugs. Both group of patients were given 100 mg LAM daily, while those in the LAM/Lingzhi group were given 50g Lingzhi and 10g red dates in addition to LAM. After 18 months, HBeAg negative converse rate and HBeAg/anti-HBe seroconversion rate in the LAM/Lingzhi group were higher than LAM group ($P < 0.05$) (Table 9-3). The HBV DNA negative converse rates in the LAM/Lingzhi group were 50/63, 56/63, 59/63 and 57/63 in 3, 6, 12 and 18 months, respectively, while those in the LAM group were 43/63, 50/63, 48/63 and 42/63 during the same periods. Lingzhi supplement showed significantly better results than LAM alone ($P < 0.05$). In LAM group, the incidence rates of the YMDD mutation, which involves tyrosine, methionine, aspartate and aspartate, of the gene that encodes the DNA sequence of the virus DNA polymerase were 11.59%, 23.81% and 33.33% in 6, 12 and 18 months, respectively. In the LAM/Lingzhi group, the rates of mutation incidence were 0, 6.35% and 9.52 % in 6, 12 and 18 months, respectively. Thus, when LAM and Lingzhi in combination was administered the mutation rate was significantly lower than when LAM was used alone (P <0. 05).

Table 9-3 HBeAg negative conversion rates (NCR) and HBeAg/HBeAb seroconversion rates (SCR) in LAM and LAM/ Lingzhi groups

Groups	Cases	Index	Post-treatment Time, month (%)			
			3	6	12	18
LAM	63	HBeAg NCR	3(4.76)	5(7.94)	8(12.70)	10(15.87)
		HBeAg/HBeAb SCR	2(3.17)	4(6.35)	8(12.70)	9(14.29)
LAM/ Lingzhi	63	HBeAg NCR	5(7.94)	11(17.46)	21(33.33)	27(42.86)
		HBeAg/HBeAb SCR	3(4.76)	7(11.11)	16(25.40)	26(41.27)

Zhong, J.P., Li, S.F. Therapeutic observation of lamivudine combined with *Ganodema japonice* for chronic hepatitis B. Modern Practical Medicine, 2006, 18(7):466-467

 Mechanism of Lingzhi's liver-protective effect

How does Lingzhi cure hepatitis? The therapeutic mechanism has been clearly elucidated by a large number of pharmacological studies. Toxic chemicals, such as carbon tetrachloride, dl-ethionine and D-galactosamine can rapidly produce toxic hepatitis in experimental animals. Other than obvious liver dysfunctions, such as ALT activity increase, there are also typical pathohistology changes in the infected liver. Administration of the extract from Lingzhi fruiting body, mycelium or spores can improve the liver function and alleviate the pathological changes in experimental animal. Lingzhi polysaccharides have been found to prevent hepatic fibrosis in experimental animals as well. The triterpenes extracted from the fruiting body are the important active ingredient for liver protection. In addition to their significant protection on the liver against damage by CCl_4 or D-galactosamine in mice, the triterpenes also play a important role in protecting the liver from immunological injury induced by Bacille Calmette-Guerin (BCG) and lipopolysac-charide (LPS) in mice. Table 9-4 shows the significant ALT and trigly-ceride (TG) reductions in the mouse liver damaged by BCG and LPS resulted from the total triterpenoid (GT) and triterpenoid composition (GT_2). The effective GT_2 dose was much lower than Malotilate, which

Table 9-4 Effect of Lingzhi triterpenoid on ALT, TG and NO in BCG and LPS induced hepatic injury in mice

Groups	Dose, mg/kg	ALT(U/L)	TG(mg/kg)	NO(μ mol/L)
Control	–	124.65±11.91	14.2±1.8	15.58±3.08
BCG+LPS	–	653.85±30.22[2]	30.2±4.2[2]	27.34±7.38[1]
BCG+LPS+Sal	–	659.78±38.38[2]	31.5±4.6[2]	28.43±7.30[1]
BCG+LPS+Mal	91	189.21±20.48[4]	15.1±2.3[4]	18.44±6.01
BCG+LPS+GT	80	318.63±31.65[3]	19.5±2.1[4]	19.48±7.99
BCG+LPS+GT$_2$	10	243.56±26.58[4]	20.5±2.8[4]	20.71±8.39
BCG+LPS+GT$_2$	20	209.41±26.88[4]	15.3±1.5[4]	18.48±5.82
BCG+LPS+GT$_2$	40	226.17±29.19[4]	18.9±2.9[4]	23.51±6.43

Sal=solvent; Mal=Malotilate(positive control drug);n=9, x s; 1) $P<0.05$; 2) $P<0.01$,compared with control; 3) $P<0.05$; 4) $P<0.01$,compare with BCG+LPS group.

is commonly used to clinically treat chronic hepatitis. Lingzhi triter-penoids have also been found to reduce nitrogen monoxide (NO) in the immunologically injured liver in mice.

The liver protective effect of Lingzhi triterpenoids is attributed to their antioxidation activity. They can not only reduce the lipid peroxi-dation product, malondialdehyde (MDA), but also increase the liver superoxide dismutase (SOD) activity and glutathione content in experi-mental mice with liver damage.

Wang, M.Y., Liu, Q., Che, Q.M. and Lin, Z.B. Effects of total triter-penoids extract from *Ganoderma lucidum* (curt.: fr.) p. karst.(reishi mushroom) on experimental liver injury models induced by carbon tetrachloride or d-galactosamine in mice. International Journal of Medi-cinal Mushrooms, 2002, 4:337-342;

Wang, M.Y., Liu, Q., Che, Q.M . and Lin, Z.B. Effects of triterpenoids from *Ganoderma lucidum* (leyss. Ex fr.) karst on three different experi-mental liver injury models in mice. Acta Pharm Sin, 2000 , 35:326-329

Can Lingzhi triterpenes inhibit hepatitis virus?

Li and Wang (2006) studied the anti-hepatitis B (anti-HBV) activity of ganoderic acid, which was one of the triterpenoids extracted from Lingzhi culture medium. The HepG2215 cell line was used in the experi-ment. The cell line, which was originated from HepG2 cell that had been infected with HBV DNA, could express HBVsurface antigen (HbsAg), core antigen (HbeAg) and the structural proteins of HBV virions, as well as reliably produce HBV mature virions. The results indicated that ganoderic acid inhibited replication of HbsAg(20%)and HBVe(44%) both dose-dependently (1-8μg/ml) and time-dependently (4 and 8 day). It was concluded that ganoderic acid inhibited hepatitis B (HBV) repli-cation, and that it was not toxic to the hepatic cells (Table 9-5).

Table9-5 Inhibition on hepatitis virus antigen and cytotoxicity to HepG 2215 cells of ganoderic acid

Dose µg/ml	Inhibition Ratio on HbsAg(%)		Inhibition Ratio on HbeAg(%)		Cytotoxicity Rate %
	4days	8days	4days	8days	
0.5	19	4	22	49	0
1	42	28	46	43	0
2	67	39	60	47	0
4	74	59	74	48	0
8	87	80	89	56	13

Li, Y.Q. and Wang, S.F. Anti-hepatitis B activities of ganoderic acid from *Ganoderma lucidum*. 2006, Biotechnol Letter, 28(11):837-841

The immunoregulating activity of Lingzhi is also involved in the mechanism of the prevention and treatment of hepatitis. Lingzhi enhances the functions of mononuclear macrophages, NK cells and T, B lymph-ocytes. It also promotes the synthesis and release of cellular immune factors, such as interleukin-2 (IL-2) and interferonγ (IFNγ). Therefore, through the intervention of Lingzhi, the immune dysfunctions caused by hepatitis may be corrected, and hepatitis viruses annihilated by the immunological cells and/or cytokine, such as IFNγ.

Chapter 10

Adjuvant Therapy for Cancers with Lingzhi

Author's prompt: Evaluation of Lingzhi in tumor therapy has been of great concern among the scientists and patients. Well controlled clinical trials showed the evidence of Lingzhi's adjuvant effects when it was applied to supplement chemotherapy or radiotherapy. These effects include reduction of bone marrow suppression, gastrointestinal injury and immunological suppression, improvement of patient's quality of life, enhancement of treatment efficacy and minimization of toxicity from the drug and radiotherapy. It is not recommended for patients to either replace the conventional therapy or use Lingzhi as the sole remedy.

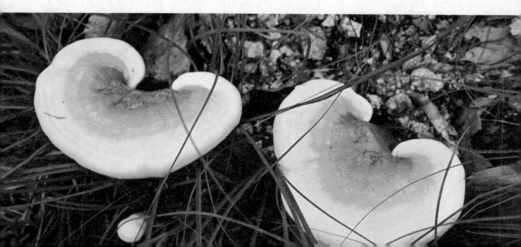

Lingzhi as an adjuvant therapy for cancers

Clinical trials on patients with cancers of the esophagus, stomach, colon, lung, liver, bladder, kidney, prostate and uterus showed desirable effects when Lingzhi preparations were administered in combination with chemotherapy or radiotherapy. Observed therapeutic improvements associated with the side effects induced by chemotherapy or radiotherapy included: (a) reduction of myelosuppression, such as leucopenia and thrombocytopenia, (b) attenuation of gastrointestinal injury, such as anorexia, nausea and vomiting, (c) enhancement of patient's immunological functions of anti-infection and anti-cancer, and (d) improvement of cancer patient's physical fitness and quality of life. The results clearly demonstrated Lingzhi's adjuvant efficacy in treating cancer patients by strengthening the immunity and decreasing toxic side effects caused by drugs or radiotherapy.

Clinical reports on Lingzhi's adjuvant treatments for cancers

Wang et al (1999) used Lingzhi decoction alone in the treatment of 22 patients of malignant neoplastic diseases. Among the 16 cases with pathological diagnosis, 8 were squamous lung cancer, 5 infiltrating type breast cancer, 2 colon adenocarcinoma and 1 small cell lung cancer. The remaining 6 cases had clinically diagnosed primary hepatic carcinoma. The 14 male and 8 female patients ranged from 41-year-old to 70-year-old (average 60). None of the patients received chemotherapy or radiotherapy, nor any treatment of biological response modifier one month prior to the trial. No biological response modification or TCM other than Lingzhi was used simultaneously during the treatment. Patients were administered Lingzhi decoction, which was made with 50 g dry Lingzhi fruiting body simmered in 500 ml water for 30 minutes, twice a day for four weeks. The following immunological indicators were compared before and after the medication: T cell subpopulation (CD3, CD4 and CD8), NK cell activity, interleukin-2 (IL-2) activity, phagocytic function (phagocytic index and rate), tumor necrosis factor (TNF), lymphocyte transformation rate, tumor marker enzyme γ -glutamyltranspeptidase (γ -GT), hepatic and renal function, blood tests (white blood cell count, platelet count and hemoglobin), one or more of the imaging diagnostic methods (computed tomography, magnetic resonance imaging and B-ultrasound), as well as patient' s complaint of symptoms and signs. The curative effects were rated according to WHO criteria with classifications of CR (complete remission, i.e., complete disappearance of visible lesions for longer than 4 weeks), PR (partial remission, i.e., tumor diminutive by more than 50% exceeding 4 weeks), MR (minor remission, i.e., tumor diminutive by more than 25%, but less than 50%, with no new lesions), SD (stable disease, i.e., tumor diminutive by less than 25% or increased by no more than 25%, with no new lesions) and PD (progressive disease, i.e., tumor increased by more than 25%, or with onset of new lesions).

After the treatment, there were 1 CR, 2 PRs, 4 MRs, 14 SDs and 1 PD. The effective rate (CR+PR) constituted 13.16% of the patients. The case of CR had a right pleural metastasis with small pleural fluids after resection of colon adenocarcinoma. Pleural fluids disappeared in the patient after one month's treatment with Lingzhi decoction, and no recurrence was observed 4 weeks afterward. As far as the quality of life is concerned, the Karnofsky score system was used for the evaluation. It was found that the scores in 8 cases (i.e., 36.4%) increased more than

10 points, those in 2 cases (i.e., 9.1%) decreased more than 10 points, and 7 cases (i.e., 31.8%) reported alleviation in generalized acratia. There were no gastrointestinal reactions, such as nausea and vomiting, observed. Nor were there any hepatic or renal dysfunction found. The white blood cells, hemoglobin and platelet counts of the patients did not decline after treatment either.

Statistically, CD3, CD4, CD4/CD8, NK cell activity, lymphocyte transformation rate and IL-2 activity increased, while CD8 decreased significantly after treatment with Lingzhi. The results indicated that Lingzhi improved the anti-tumor immunity of the patients. The phagocytic index, phagocytic rate and TNF increased slightly, but not significantly different from pre-treatment data. γ-GT is a tumor marker enzyme reflecting the degree of cellular canceration. Its up-regulation often correlates with the canceration progress. In the trial, γ-GT content in the patients dropped from 101.03 ±17.79 IU/L to 70.65 ±15.05 IU/L with the Lingzhi treatment. Declining γ-GT activity in cancer tissue and serum suggested that Lingzhi might redirect the cancer cells to become normal and reverse the canceration process.

The authors postulated that the reason for the low effective rate, 13.6%, was due to the fact that the size of the tumor masses was beyond the killing range of zero-order kinetic immunotherapy. However, immunotherapy is the only remaining option for treating the residual cancer cells or micrometastasis after surgical resection, radiotherapy or chemotherapy. Consequently, it was concluded that supplementing surgery, radiotherapy and/or chemotherapy with Lingzhi could provide a synergistic anti-tumor effect.

Wang, H.J., Liu, Y.E., Chen, J. et al. Clinical research of decoction of *Ganoderma lucidum* on treatment of malignant tumors. Journal of Dalian

Medical University, 1999,21(1):29-31

Yan et al (1998) investigated the clinical efficacy of Lingzhi oral liquid (an extract of the fruiting body) combined with chemotherapy in 56 cases of advanced non-small cell lung cancer. The 29 male and 27 female patients averaged 56.2-year-old. The patients were diagnosed with highly suspected clinical manifestations and epidemiological chara-cteristics of lung cancer, confirmed by chest radiology and computed tomography (CT) tests, and histopathology or cytological examination with primary non-small cell lung cancer. The patients were unable or unwilling to be subjected to surgery, or had postoperative intrapulmonary recurrence that had disseminated. They were otherwise in generally good condition with Karnofsky score greater than 60 and an expected survival time more than 3 months. All patients had their lesion shown on X-ray, CT or magnetic resonance imaging (MRI) for size determina-tion. All 56 lung cancer patients were in II to IV stage, including 26 in II and III stages and 30 in III and IV stages. There were 32 cases of lung adenocarcinoma, 15 cases of squamous cell carcinoma, 7 cases of squa-mous adenocarcinoma and 2 cases of large cell carcinoma.

The patients were randomly divided, 35 in Treatment Group (Ling-zhi oral liquid+ chemotherapy) and 21 in the Control Group (chemo-therapy only). Before the treatment, the Karnofsky scores of the Treatment and the Control Groups averaged 60.5 and 70, respectively, with no significant differences in their disease conditions. Three times a day, 20ml of Lingzhi oral liquid was administered for a month. Prescription of cisplatin (DDP) plus vindesine (VDS) for chemotherapy was applied in the following manner: for the Treatment Group, 40 mg DDP and 500ml saline by intravenous drip for 5 days, followed by a 20 day interval before the second monthly treatment [Note: VDS dosage and application were not specified in the report]. At the same time, Lingzhi oral liquid was given to the patients in the Treatment Group. The treatment efficacy was evaluated after 2 consecutive monthly treatments. Short-term curative effect was classified based on the WHO objective evaluation criteria of solid tumor as: complete remission (CR), partial remission (PR), minor remission (MR), stable disease (SD), MR+SD for no change (NC) and progressive disease (PD). The effective rate (CR+PR) was the remission rate (RR). Change in patient's quality of life, based on Karnofsky score, was classified as "improvement" when the score increased less than 10, "stabilization"when no change occurred, and "decline" when reduced more than 10. Counts on red blood cells (RBC), white blood cells (WBC), hemoglobin (HGB), platelets (PLT), T lymphocytes and T lymphocytes subsets were determined. Data from the patients, who completed the two monthly treatments, were used for statistical analysis. Those from the patients, who discontinued or died during the course, were counted as invalid (PD).

The results are as follows: 2 CRs (i.e., 5.7% of the total), 21 PRs (i.e., 60%), 9 NCs (i.e., 25.71%), 3 PDs (i.e., 8.57%) and 23 CR+PR (i.e., 65.71%) from the Treatment Group; and, 1 CR (i.e., 4.76%),8 PRs (i.e., 38.14%), 10 NCs (i.e., 47.62%), 2 PDs (i.e., 9.52%) and 9 CR+PR (i.e., 42.85%) from the Control Group. Comparing RR of the Treatment and the Control Groups, there was a significant difference (P<0.01).

The Karnofsky scores showed 24 "improvements" (i.e., 68.57%), 7 "stabilizations"(i.e., 20%) and 4 "declines"(i.e., 11.43%) in the Treatment Group; and, in the Control Group, 9 "improvements" (i.e., 42.85%), 8 "stabilizations"(i.e., 38.10%) and 4 "declines"(i.e., 19.05%). The improvement rate in the Treatment Group, 68.57%, was significantly higher than that in the Control Group (i.e., 42.85%) (P<0.01). Meanwhile, the life quality improvement rate in the Treatment Group was greater than the remission rate suggesting that even though patients might not have achieved CR or PR, their quality of life materially improved.

Hematology tests did not show apparent changes in patients in the Treatment Group after the trial. On the other hand, the RBC, WBC, HGB and PLT counts in the Control Group decreased significantly. This indicated that the Lingzhi oral liquid lessened the suppression on the bone marrow hematopoietic function induced by the chemotherapy.

In varying degrees, T3, T4 and T8 in the Treatment Group increased significantly after the treatment. Whereas, they decreased in the Control Group, although statistically insignificant. The results suggest that Lingzhi might enhance the cellular immune function in cancer patients.

Yan, B.K., Wei, Y.J. and Li, Y.Q. Clinical observation of Lingzhi oral liquid combined with chemotherapy in 56 cases of advanced non-small cell lung cancer. Traditional Chinese Drug Research & Clinical Pharmacology, 1998, 9(2): 78-80

Lin et al (2004) compared the effect of Lingzhi extract combined with chemotherapy on 114 cases of cancer patients. These patients were confirmed with cancers of the stomach, esophagus, lung, liver, cervix, colon or bladder by pathological, cytological and CT examination, based on the *National Guidelines for Diagnosis and Treatment of the Common Cancers in China* (WHO, 1979). All patients were randomly divided into two groups, i.e., "chemotherapy with Lingzhi group (CL)" (66 cases) and "chemotherapy control group (CC)" (48 cases). In CC, the FAM chemotherapy was applied, including intravenous injections of 300 mg/m² 5-flurouracil twice a week and 30 mg/m² adriamycin once a week in the first and the fourth weeks, and bolus intravenous injection of 3mg/m² mitomycin once a week, for 6 weeks as one course of treatment. After

4 to 5 months, the treatment could be repeated according to the patients' conditions. For the patients in CL, in addition to the same chemotherapy, 4 capsules of Lingzhi fruiting body extract were administered, 4 times daily for 40 days as one course of treatment.

The results demonstrated that Lingzhi extract markedly ameliorated immune suppression induced by chemotherapy. In CL, the natural killer cells (NK) activities in the patients were 51.24±7.9 before, and 48.10 ±7.90 after the treatment, showing no statistically significant difference (P> 0.05). On the other hand, those in CC were 51.40±6.62 before, and 44.43±7.19 after the treatment, showing a statistically significant difference (P<0.05). As shown in Table 10-1, the CD3, CD4 and CD8 cell subsets in CL changed little, but in CC, they were significantly depressed by the treatment. Further more, both clinical symptoms and quality of life of the patients in CL were improved.

Lin, N.D., Su, J.N., Gao, Y.H. et al. Clinical analysis of 66 cases of treatment with *Ganoderma lucidum* extract combined chemotherapy for tumors. Journal of Practical Traditional Chinese Internal Medicine, 2004, 18(5):457-458

Table 10-1 Change in percentage on T-lymphocyte subsets in CL and CC groups before and after treatments

Groups	N		CD_3	CD_4	CD_8
CL	66	Before	51.43± 6.00	36.57± 6.69	31.20± 6.90
		After	5 0.67± 6.29	37.10± 6.49	30.24± 7.60
CC	48	Before	50.99± 6.52	37.75± 7.40	30.99± 6.69
		After	43.38± 6.39*	31.01± 6.31*	26.42± 7.15*

$\bar{x}±s$;$^*P$ <0.05, compared with before and after the treatment in the same group.

Ni et al (1997) conducted a clinical study using Lingzhi spore powder capsules on cancer patients. These patients had been diagnosed with "deficiencies in the spleen" according to TCM practice, and were receiving radiotherapy and chemotherapy. A total of 160 participating outpatients and inpatients were randomized divided into Test (50 patients were receiving chemotherapy and 50 radiotherapy) and Control (30 were receiving chemotherapy and 30 radiotherapy) Groups. There were no significant differences on gender and age between the two groups. The symptoms of "deficiencies in the spleen" included anorexia, fatigue/hypologia, lassitude, abdominal distention, loose stool, pale complexion, thin muscles, pale tongue and weak pulse. All patients exhibited the first 3 major symptoms, in addition to the tongue or pulse diagnostic judgment. In Test Group, 69%-87% of the patients had anorexia, fatigue/hypologia and lassitude, while in the Control Group, 76.7%-80%. All of the 160 cancer cases were confirmed by imaging and pathocytological diagnosis with 12 types of tumors on the esophagus, lung or breast. There was no significant difference on the cancer type distribution between the Test and the Control Group. Patients, who did not meet the abovementioned criteria, had heart, brain, lung, liver, kidney and hematopoietic complications, or did not comply with the medication regiments were excluded from the trial. Starting 3 days before radiotherapy or chemotherapy, patients in the Test Group were given oral administration of 0.4g Lingzhi spore powder capsules, 3 times a day for one month as one course of treatment. Patients in the Control Group received their regular radiotherapy or chemotherapy without the Lingzhi capsules during the same time period.

Clinical observations of changes in the symptom of "deficiencies in the spleen" and tongue/pulse appearances were conducted and used for grading according to TCM methodology. Patient's quality of life was estimated by using the Karnofsky score system. The peripheral white blood cell, lymphocyte and platelet counts, as well as the immunoglobulin test were also determined on patients before and after the treatment. The criteria and classification for the clinical efficacy included: (a) excellence, i.e., marked improvement on symptoms was evident, the symptom grading scale decreased equal or more than 2/3 of the pre-treatment score, Karnofsky score increased 30 points, and the laboratory analyses ameliorated by 11%-20%; (b) effective, i.e., improvement on symptoms was evident, the symptom grading scale decreased equal or more than 1/3 of the pre-treatment score, Karnofsky score increased 10 points, and the laboratory analyses ameliorated by 5%-10%; and, (c) failure, i.e., no improvement of symptoms observed, the symptom grading scale decreased less than 1/3 of the pre-treatment score, had no increase in Karnofsky scores, and no apparent change on laboratory data was found.

Comparing the patients in the Test Group to those in the Control Group, the Karnofsky score was 91.0% vs. 30.0%; the TCM grading scales was 86.0% vs. 26.7%, the average effective rate according to the improvement of five major symptoms on the "deficiencies in the spleen" beyond (+) was 73.9% vs. 15.8%; the average effective rate according to the improvement of the first 3 major symptoms of the "deficiencies in the spleen" was 87.4% vs. 26.3% (Table 10-2). There are significant differences on all indices between the Test and the Control Group. The white blood cell count and hemoglobin content in the two groups also changed significantly before and after the treatment (Table 10-3).

Ni, J.Y., Wang, X.M. and He, W.Y. Clinical study of efficacy of *Ganoderma lucidum* spore powder capsules on cancer patients with "deficiencies in the spleen" receiving radiotherapy and chemotherapy. Clinical

Journal of Anhui Traditional Chinese Medicine, 1997, 9(6): 292-293

Table 10-2 Curative effects based on symptom improvements on patients

Symptoms	Test Group		Control Group	
	cases	Effective	cases	Effective
Anorexia	69	61(88.4%)	46	14(30.4%)
Fatigue/hypología	87	79(90.8%)	48	11(22.9%)
Lassitude	83	69(83.1%)	47	12(25.5%)
Abdominal distension	12	6(50.0%)	6	0(0)
Loose stool	14	8(57.1%)	7	0(0)

Table 10-3 Hematological changes on patients before and after treatment ($\bar{x}$ ± s)

	Index	Groups	n	before	after	difference
Lung cancer	WBC(10^9/L)	Test	10	3.93± 0.48	4.77± 0.43	0.76± 0.53
		Control	9	4.59± 0.36	4.00± 0.15	-0.70± 0.29
	Hb(g/L)	Test	10	8.53± 1.67	9.72± 1.24	1.08± 0.75
		Control	9	8.00± 0.66	7.33± 1.17	-0.89± 0.22
Esophageal and gastric carcinoma	WBC(10^9/L)	Test	10	3.83± 0.50	4.90± 0.82	1.07± 0.93
		Control	10	4.45± 1.04	3.62± 0.49	-0.85± 0.94
	Hb(g/L)	Test	10	8.23± 1.67	10.08± 8.91	1.85± 0.86
		Control	10	8.15± 1.67	6.26± 10.21	-1.89± 1.92

Zhou et al (2001) reported the role of Lingzhi teabag in adjuvant therapy for tumors. In the study, 309 patients with confirmed cases of advanced malignant tumors were included. Of which, 155 cases were placed in the Treatment Group, and 154 in Control Group. Prior to the admission, the patient's general conditions, total white blood cell count, granulocyte count, appetite and chemotherapy were similar for the two groups. The chemotherapy also included anti-emetic drugs and leucocyte increasing agents (leucogen and Batilol tablets). In the Treatment Group, patients were given Lingzhi teabags containing diced fruiting body for administration starting 3 days before chemotherapy. For the following 15-20 days, 2-4 g of the teabag was used, twice a day, for each patient. The efficacy criteria included: (1) nausea and vomiting: "0"for none, "I"for vomiting 1-2 times, and"II"for vomiting 3-4 times, "III"for vomiting more than 5 times a day; (2) food intake: "I"for eating nothing or less than half of normal amount, "II"for eating half of the normal amount, and"III"for normal consumption; and, (3) peripheral blood test conducted every 3 days, 3-4 times before and after chemotherapy.

After the chemotherapy, the nausea and vomiting ratings among the patients in the Treatment Group were 59 of "0",77 of "I",16 of "II" and 3 of "III", while those in the Control Group were 31, 92, 25 and 6, respectively. Food intakes of the patients in the Treatment Group were 17 of "I", 81 of "II"and 57 of "III",while those in the Control Group were 39, 74 and 41, respectively. Decreases in WBC among patients in the Treatment Group were less than those in the Control Group. The results showed that administration of Lingzhi tea relieved vomiting and improved appetite for patients after chemotherapy, that is, Lingzhi plays an adjuvant role in the cancer treatment.

Zhou, J., Zou, X.X. and Zhou, J.C. Clinical observation of *Ganoderma lucidum* preparation in adjuvant therapy for tumors. Jiangxi Journal of Traditional Chinese Medicine, 2001, 32(3): 30,32

Mechanism of anti-tumor activity of Lingzhi in adjuvant therapy

Pharmacological studies have demonstrated that oral or injection of Lingzhi extract, or ganoderma polysaccharides, exhibited significant anti-tumor effect in tumor-bearing animals. However, they can by no means kill the tumor cells, nor promote apoptosis in vitro. The fact suggests that Lingzhi extract and polysaccharides are not cytotoxic to tumor cells. Then, how does the anti-tumor effect occur in tumor-bearing animals in vivo? It has been proven that ganoderma polysaccharides have immunomodulatory activity, including enhancing the maturation and function of dendritic cells, increasing activities of macrophages, the natural killer cells (NK) and cytotoxic T cell, modulating humoral and cellular immunity, and promoting secretion of anti-tumor cytokines, such as tumor necrosis factor (TNF) and interferon (IFN). Therefore, the anti-tumor efficacy of Lingzhi water extract, or the polysaccharides, was mainly a result of their immunostimulating activity. On the other hand, it differs from the polysaccharides, the triterpene fraction of Lingzhi has been reported with in vitro anti-tumor activity.

Lingzhi has also been found to inhibit tumor angiogenesis. Angiogenesis, i.e., the formation of blood vessels by capillaries sprouting from pre-existing vessels, provides nutrition for cellular growth. It is an important normal physiological function, and at the same time, it can become pathological in the cases, such as tumor growth and metastasis. Pharmacological studies have confirmed that ganoderma polysaccharides' in vivo anti-angiogenesis activity can directly inhibit proliferation of the human umbilical vein endothelial cells (HUVEC). Thereby, the resulting endothelial cell apoptosis depletes blood and nutrient supply to the tumor causing its growth retardation.

Li et al. (2008) investigated the effect of ganoderma polysaccharides (*Gl*-PS) on reversing multi-drug resistance (MDR) of the adriamycin-resistant leukemic cell line K562/ADM. Results indicated that *Gl*-PS significantly reversed K562/ADM's resistance to adriamycin (doxorubicin) by down-regulating the expression of MDR-1 and MDR-associated protein (MRP). MDR is a major cause of cancer treatment failure, due to cancer cell's developing resistance to a wide variety of chemotherapeutic drugs. It has been associated with the overexpression of P-glycoprotein (P-gp) or MRP, which are two transmembrane transporters that act as pumps to remove toxic drugs from tumor cells. This mechanism might attribute to Lingzhi's synergic effect with chemotherapy.

Li, W.D., Zhang, B.D., Wei, R. et al. Reversal effect of *Ganoderma lucidum* polysaccharide on multidrug resistance in K562/ADM cell line. Acta Pharmacol Sin, 2008 , 29 (5): 620-627

Another pharmacological study reported the anti-radiation effect of Lingzhi (Fig. 10-1). It reduced the gastrointestinal injury induced by radiation or chemotherapy, enhanced anti-tumor effects of the chemotherapeutant, such as cyclophosphamide, fluorouracil, doxorubicin, cisplatin and Ara-C, and relieved the immunosuppression or myelosuppression induced by mitomycin C, fluorouracil and Ara-C (Table 10-4, 5). These findings are in agreement with the clinical observations of the adjuvant effects of Lingzhi.

Furusawa E, Chou SC, Furusawa S, et al. Antitumor activity of *Ganokerma lucidum*, an edible mushroom, on interaperitoneally implanted lewis lung carcinoma in synergenic mice. Phytotherapy Res, 1992, 6: 300~304

Lei, LS, Lin, ZB, Chen, Q, et al. Antagonistic effect of *Ganoderma lucidum* polyscharides on the immunosuppressive response induced by ciclosporin A, hydrocortisone and antitumor agents. Chin J Pharmacol Toxicol, 1993, 7(3):183-185

TCM therapeutical theory of "strengthening health to ward off invading pathogens" and Lingzhi's adjuvant therapy for tumors

Tumors can be removed by surgery and cancerous cells diminished or eliminated by chemotherapy or radiotherapy. However, there is no guarantee for complete avoidance of tumor metastasis or residual tumor cells after the treatments. Moreover, damages caused by surgery and toxicities induced by chemotherapy or radiotherapy can depress the body's immunity to fight against tumors. In fact, death can result directly or

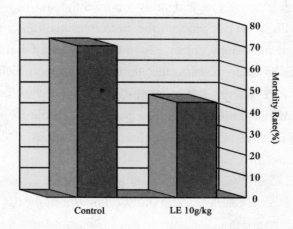

Fig. 10-1 Effect of Lingzhi extract (LE) on mouse mortality in 30 days after ^{60}Co-ray irradiation

Table 10-4 Effect of Lingzhi extract (LE) combined with cytotoxic anti-neoplastics on Lewis lung sarcoma in mice

Drug(s) Applied	Dose, i.p.	Life Span	Survivals	Life Extension Rate
Control		13.4± 2.9	0/10	
LE	10 mg, 2,4,6,8,10 day	25.5± 8.0**	0/10	90
Doxorubicin		22.6± 7.8**	1/10	67
LE + Doxorubicin	See above	36.5± 6.9++	7/10	172
Control		11.8± 3.0	0/5	
LE	10 mg, 2,4,6,8,10 day	23.8± 4.4**	0/5	102
Cisplatin	5 mg, 1 day	18.8± 5.3*	0/5	59
LE + Cisplatin	See above	35.6± 5.4++	2/5	202
Control		14.8± 3.3	0/10	
LE	10 mg, 2,4,6,8,10 day	26.3± 7.2**	1/10	78
Fluorouracil	0.3 mg, 1 day	26.5± 7.1**	0/10	79
LE + Fluorouracil	See above	34.4± 8.5+	6/10	132
Control		17.6± 3.1	0/10	
LE	10 mg, 2,4,6,8,10 day	28.2± 7.6**	2/10	60
Tioguanine	0.1 mg, 1 day	25.5± 6.4**	0/10	49
LE + Tioguanine	See above	36.2± 6.3++	7/10	106
methopterin	0.2 mg, 1 day	24.2± 4.8*	0/5	38
LE + methopterin	See above	36.6± 46.5+	3/6	106

$^*P<0.05$, $^{**}P<0.01$, compared with control group; $^+P<0.05$, $^{++}P<0.01$, compared with monotherapy

Table 10-5 Recovery effect of ganoderma polysaccharides （GL-B）on suppression of mixed lymphocyte reaction （MLR）induced by mitomycin C, fluorouracil and cytarabine

Groups	Concentration (μg/ml)	[³H]TdR uptake (dpm)
Control	—	31361± 4242
Mitomycin C (positive control)	0.01	16842± 1266+++
Mitomycin C+GL-B	0.01+50	19003± 978**
Mitomycin C+GL-B	0.01+100	24209± 1505***
Mitomycin C+GL-B	0.01+200	27606± 2372***
Control	—	28946± 1527
5-fluorouracil (positive control)	0.1	16250± 1614+++
5-fluorouracil + GL-B	0.1+50	20875± 1750***
5-fluorouracil + GL-B	0.1+100	26201± 2130***
5-fluorouracil + GL-B	0.1+200	28823± 1728***
Control	—	23678± 1348
Cytarabine (positive control)	0.1	13091± 1973+++
Cytarabine + GL-B	0.1+50	17658± 2420**
Cytarabine + GL-B	0.1+100	24380± 2949***
Cytarabine + GL-B	0.1+200	30030± 4649***

$\bar{x}$± s, n=6, +++P<0.001, compared with control group, **P<0.01, ***P<0.001, compared with positive control group.

indirectly from injuries in bone marrow, digestive system, liver, kidney and other vital organs. The "collateral damage" on healthy cells is a result of the nature of radiotherapy and chemotherapy, which do not distinguish "friends or foes" in their action on our body. In view of TCM therapeutic theory, surgical resection, chemotherapy or radiotherapy for treating tumors emphasizes "fighting against the invading pathogens". They do not strengthen the body's self-defense system to ward off the invaders. Worse yet, they weaken the power of immunity and detoxification ability of our body resulting in unexpected outcomes with the therapies. Thus, the adjunctive role of Lingzhi in supplementing cancer chemotherapy and radiotherapy fills in the gap. Lingzhi's effects in enhancing anti-tumor immunity, promoting bone marrow hematopoiesis and reducing radio-therapy or chemotherapy damages yields the end result of "strengthening health to ward off invading pathogens" as TCM theorizes. Cancer patients, who live with the tumors after Lingzhi treatment, could possibly because of their strengthened anti-tumor immunity that retards further development or metastasis of the tumors. In other words, Lingzhi empowers the body's resistance to diseases making the long-term survival possible for the cancer patients.

Finally, it cannot be over-emphasized that, despite its well-accepted anti-tumor effect, Lingzhi should not be a replacement for the conventional anti-tumor drugs and/or treatments. Lingzhi should only be recognized, and is best used, as an effective adjuvant to help improve the curing efficacy and decrease toxicity in treating cancers.

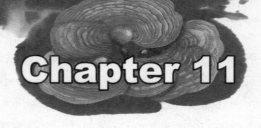

Chapter 11

Care for Health of the Sub-Healthy, Middle-Aged and Elderly

Author's prompt: The middle-aged and elderly, especially the "sub-healthy" people should take advantage of the disease preventing effect of Lingzhi for their health. Strengthening health to prevent sickness would be superior to curing a disease. Based on individual needs and physiological conditions, adequate use of Lingzhi can improve our immunity, body functions and adaptability to changes that lead to a longer lifespan and better well-being.

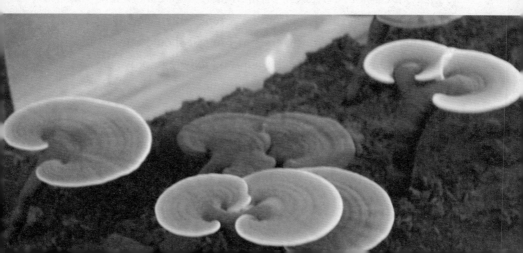

TCM emphasizes health and well-being

In the long history of medical practices, TCM developed a keen understanding of the relationship of human physiology and medication. It strongly believes in disease prevention. Long before the last century when the western medical professionals finally realized the direct association with human diet and health, statements, such as "medicine and food both affect human health" already appeared in Chinese literature. TCM defines a good physician as "one who treats an ailment before the symptom appears, and who fosters good health to prevent illness." It considers "the treatment superior if the patient is treated before sickness arrives, mediocre when a disease is emerging, and inferior for the ailment on hand." It likens physicians to politicians: "A statesman serves the country, a good doctor helps mankind, and the least desirable doctor cures diseases." These vividly display TCM's emphasis on health and well-being, and in disease prevention rather than remedy. Lingzhi was listed in the *Shennong Material Medica* as a superior medicine, which provides the effect on maintaining health without toxicity even for long-term use, as well as benefits energy and life-enhancement. It is evident that, more than 2000 years ago, TCM already recognized the healthful and anti-aging efficacies of many Chinese medicinal materials, such as Lingzhi.

 ## "Sub-health" and homeostasis regulation disorder

In 1978, the World Health Organization redefined health as more than the absence of disease or disability, but also the state of physical, mental, social and spiritual well-being. That concurred with the "biological-psychological-social" medical viewpoint evolved from the former biological model. Thereby, a "third state" between health and sickness came to being, which is now known as the "sub-health state." "Sub-health" refers to a physiological state characterized by reduced vitality and adaptability in a person. Although lacking apparent diagnostic symptoms, a large proportion of the populace belongs to the sub-health group with a feeling of physical and/or psychological inadequacies. This undesirable health condition results from disorders on the nerves-endocrine-immune regulation, physiology and metabolism. And, it is shown externally by low energy, tenseness, anxiety, insomnia, dreams, dizziness, tinnitus, nervousness, fatigue, poor appetite, weakness, etc. The furious competition, rapid living pace, lifestyle and diet changes, environmental pollution, ecological imbalance, etc. in the modern society are possible causes of this health inadequacy. As we age, the inadequate condition becomes increasingly serious, and hypertension, hyperlipemia, diabetes and/or cardiovascular diseases may develop. In addition, a lowered immunity can also increase the incidences of bacterial or viral infections and cancers.

Much earlier than the western medicine, TCM recognized the problems of sub-health. In the *Plain Questions of Huangdi's Internal Classic*

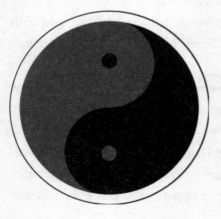

(475 – 221 B.C.) indicated that the primary purpose of medicine was "to eliminate faults before they surface" and "to gain health by healing the wounds", and that curing the disease was considered secondary. By saying "before they surface", it means that there is a lack of apparent signs of a disease, while "the wound" refers to being weak and unhealthy,

not necessarily sick. Thus, the description of what is now called "sub-health".

People in the sub-health state need to avoid further deterioration, lest he will become ill. Under normal or healthy conditions, our nerve, cardiovascular, endocrine and immune systems coordinate and function smoothly through the self-regulating and intermodulating mechanisms. The body regulates functions of these systems according to the environmental factors. For example, tension of the vascular smooth muscle can be adjusted by inputs from the sublimis sympathetic center in the brain, sympathetic nerves, renin-angiotensin system in the kidney and/or endocrine system. A normal blood pressure can thus be maintained under varying internal and external conditions. Dysfunction in the systems can lead to hypertension. Another example involves blood sugar. The insulin secreted by pancreatic islet cells (B cells) reduces the blood sugar, but the glucagon secreted by A cells increases blood sugar. Other endocrine hormones, such as adrenal cortex hormones, growth hormone and adrenaline also have antagonistic effects on the insulin causing a rise in blood sugar. However, secretions of these hormones are regulated by the nerve, endocrine and immune systems. Hence, only when all these factors are in perfect balance, can the body maintain a normal blood sugar level.

In essence, sub-health is due to a disturbance of the body's homeostasis regulation. Dysfunction on the regulation reduces the body's adaptability to internal or external changes. It may eventually lead to diseases. Consequently, normal homeostasis regulation is crucial to human health. As long as the body maintains normal regulatory functions, health can be expected.

Health effect of Lingzhi on sub-healthy populations

As we grow older, important organs in our body, such as the nerve, cardiovascular, endocrine and immune systems, begin to regress. Along with the regression process, disorders in the homeostasis regulation and adaptability to environmental changes become increasingly pronounced. The bodily deterioration makes us vulnerable to a host of diseases, such as cardiovascular, diabetes, viral infections, cancer, etc. During this time, using Lingzhi to strengthen those vital organs should be conceivably beneficial in getting the pressure, viscosity, as well as lipid and sugar contents of the blood in check. At the same time, it can enhance the immunity, improve the adaptability, delay the aging process, and prevent the diseases that commonly occur among the middle-aged and elderly. In general, the dosage of Lingzhi required for such purposes is small. Regular and continual use of Lingzhi can promote health and well-being.

 Anti-aging effect of Lingzhi

Elixir is a myth. Nonetheless, the powerful and the wealthy are after it. Their desire and pursuit of longevity may be illusive, as death is natural and inevitable. On the other hand, both scientifically and in reality, human's life expectancy should be much higher than 100 years. Delaying the aging process to achieve long life ought to be attainable. Moreover, prolonging lifespan must be accompanied by an enhanced quality of life. To that effect, "The Six Zhis" in *Shennong Materia Medica* stressed that Lingzhi relies on long-term use for its efficacy in extending life. Why, then, does Lingzhi possess the power to delay the aging process?

First of all, Lingzhi can rejuvenate the impaired immunity associated with aging. Immune function regression is the earliest and the most obvious sign of aging. The thymus, an important immune organ, begins progressive degradation at the beginning of puberty. It controls the T cell function and its cytokine producing ability. As thymus regresses with age, the immunity declines. Secondly, the B cell's immunoglobulin secretion ability, regulated by bone marrow, also decreases with age. These changes invariably lead to a weakened immunity and a reduced ability in monitoring antigen mutation. As a result, the elderly become more susceptible to infectious diseases, tumor growth and immune defi-ciency. Studies have shown that the regression of the immune functions caused by aging can be delayed and partially reversed.

Pharmacological studies have shown that Lingzhi can significantly restore the degrading of the humoral as well as the cell immune func-tions caused by aging. It can also promote cytokine production in the aging mice. As shown in Table 11-1, the spontaneous proliferation and interleukin-2 (IL-2) production by the spleen cells in the 24-month-old mice are significantly lower than those of the 3-month-old mice, decrea-sing by 27.4% and 30.1%, respectively. Ganoderma polysaccharides (GL-B) restored the levels in the aging mice to the 3-month-old mice levels, in a dose-dependent manner. Table 11-2 shows that the DNA polymerase α activity of the spleen cells in 24-month-old mice reduced by 43.3% from that of the 3-month-old mice. The result indicates that the age-related reduction of immune function is related to the DNA dysynthesis of the immune cells. Daily intra-peritoneal injection of 25 mg/kg or 50 mg/kg GL-B on the aging mice for 4 days significantly enhanced the DNA polymerase α activity of the spleen cells in the mice, and restored it to the normal level.

Furthermore, the anti-aging effect of Lingzhi is also related to its anti-oxidation and free radical scavenging abilities. Free radicals are highly active substances produced during cell metabolism. They can turn unsaturated lipids in cell membrane into peroxidized products through lipid peroxidation. Lipid peroxides (LPOs) cause changes in the cell

Table 11-1 Effects of GL-B on spontaneous proliferation and IL-2 production of spleen cells in mice

Group	Age of Mice (months)	Concentration (µg/ml)	[³H]TdR uptake × 10⁻³ (dpm)	IL-2 activity× 10⁻³ (dpm)
Young Control	3	-	45.4± 2.1	8.3± 1.4
Old Control	24	-	19.4± 3.88⁺⁺⁺	5.8± 1.0⁺
GL-B	24	50	34.8± 4.5	7.3± 1.2*
GL-B	24	100	36.1± 2.6**	8.2± 1.0**
GL-B	24	200	40.2± 4.2***	9.0± 1.0***

$\bar{x}$± s, n=6; ⁺P<0.05, ⁺⁺⁺P<0.001 compared with the Young control; *P<0.05, **P<0.01, ***P<0.001 compared with the Old control.

Table 11-2 Effects of GL-B on DNA polymerase α activity of spleen cells in mice

Group	Age of Mice (months)	Dose (mg/kg× d)	DNA Polymerase α Activity (U/10¹⁰ Spleen Cells)
Young Control	3	-	16.3± 3.2
Old Control	24	-	9.20± 2.4⁺⁺⁺
GL-B	24	25	13.3± 3.0**
GL-B	24	50	14.6± 3.6**

$\bar{x}$± s, n=6, ⁺⁺⁺P <0.001, compared with the Young control; **P <0.01, compared with the Old control.

structure and functions, resulting in damages to the organs and tissues. Under normal circumstances, the production and removal of oxygen free radicals are in balance. When over-abundant free radicals are presented or the scavenging function becomes inappropriate, the accumulated free radicals can induce detrimental effects to the body, such as damaging (1) cell lipids and membrane, (2) proteins and enzymes, and (3) nucleic acids and chromosomes. A theory on aging believes that lipid peroxidation and excessive free radicals lead to senescence of cells, tissues and organs, thus, the progress of aging process.

Pharmacological studies indicate that Lingzhi can protect against lipid peroxidation caused by a variety of factors in the heart, liver, kidney, pancreas, brain, and other vital organs. Lingzhi can significantly reduce the amount of lipid peroxidation products, such as malondialdehyde (MDA) and lipofuscin, as well as enhance the activity of antioxidative enzymes, such as superoxide dismutase (SOD) and glutathione peroxidase (GSH-PX). With the in vitro macrophages (mouse), islet cells (mouse), cerebral cortex cells (rat), PC12 cells (i.e., rat pheochromocytoma cells, which are widely used culture model for investigations on neuron development and functions of various diseases, such as the Parkinson's, Alzheimer's), vascular endothelial cells (rat and human) and keratinocytes (human), Lingzhi has demonstrated a significant protective effect against the oxidant-induced oxidative damage. In Table 11-3, it shows that after hydrogen peroxide (H_2O_2), a cell-aging inducing agent, was placed 3 times on cultured human keratinocytes, the cell debris increased as observed under the microscope. At the same time, MDA began to accumulate in cells, while SOD, GSH-PX and other antioxidative enzyme levels reduced. These are signs of premature senility. By application of 400 μg/ml GL-B before hydrogen peroxide, the oxidative damage on the human keratinocytes was significantly repaired. The polysaccharides can also reduce MDA formation in normal keratinocytes. Keratinocytes are major epidermal cells. Their deterioration directly reflects aging of the skin. Thus, the results suggest that Lingzhi may have a cosmetic effect for skin care.

Reports on the health effects of Lingzhi

Enhance immunity among the elderly

Tao and Ye (1993) studied the effect of Lingzhi on the cellular immune function on 30 cases of elderly subjects. Healthy volunteers, 19 males and 11 females with an average age of 65.1, participated in the trial. Among them, 13 had high blood lipids (i.e., cholesterol > 6.0 mmol/L, triglycerides > 1.25 mmol/L and LDL-cholesterol > 5.8mmol/L) and 21 had cerebral arteriosclerosis. None used TCM herbs, glucocorticoids or other drugs, which could affect the immune function, in 6 months prior to the trial. They were given 1.5 g Lingzhi powder 3 times

Table 11-3 In vitro effects of GL-B on activity of SOD and GSH-PX, and MDA in human keratinocytes damaged by hydrogen peroxide

Group	SOD (U/ml)	GSH-PX (U)	MDA (nmol/mg protein)
Control	40.22± 3.32	202.11± 19.89	1.56± 0.17
H_2O_2	21.54± 2.33*	120.55± 13.34*	2.55± 0.26*
GL-B + H_2O_2	35.76± 3.45△	188.66± 17.76△	1.87± 0.16△
GL-B	42.91± 1.53	214.00± 23.23	1.12± 0.10*

$\bar{x}\pm s$, *$P<0.05$, compared with the Control; $P<0.05$, GL-B+H_2O_2 compared with H_2O_2 Group.

a day for 30 days. On the 10th, 20th and 30th day after the beginning of the administration, as well as the 10th day after stopping the administration, vein blood samples were collected from all participants. The peripheral blood mononuclear cells were isolated and IL-2, IFNγ and NK activity determined. The results (Table 11-4) showed that IL-2, IFNγ levels and NK activity increased, reaching a peak at the 20th day of Lingzhi administration. The peaked activities remained 10 days after stopping the treatment. It is, therefore, concluded that Lingzhi can improve immunity for the elderly.

Table 11-4 Effects of Lingzhi powder on IL-2 and IFNγ and NK in the elderly

Time of Sampling	IL-2 (U/ml)	IFNγ (U/ml)	NK (%)
Before drug administration	134.1± 30.7	8.3± 3.9	40.1± 10.3
Drug administration for 10 days	150.7± 41.3**	10.6± 4.3*	48.7± 9.6**
Drug administration for 20 days	159.2± 39.4**	11.5± 5.2**	51.3± 9.1**
Drug administration for 30 days	154.8± 36.7**	11.9± 5.6**	50.7± 8.4**
10 days after drug withdrawal	157.8± 41.9**	12.1± 5.9**	50.1± 9.3**

$\bar{x}±$ s; *$P<0.05$, **$P<0.01$ compared with sampling before drug administration

Tao, S.X. and Ye, C.S. Effect of *Ganoderma lucidum* on cellular immune function of the elderly. Chinese Journal of Geriatrics, 1993, 12: 298-301

Treatment for male menopause syndrome

The menopause symptoms between male and female are very similar. Besides reduction of androgen, the body metabolism (e.g., microcirculation, free radical oxygen balance, blood viscosity, etc.) goes through noticeable changes at the same time. They invariably affect the aging process.

The following 3 clinical reports illustrate how the sporoderm-broken Lingzhi spores improved the male menopause syndrome, and Lingzhi methanol or ethanol extract ameliorated the urinary symptoms of benign prostatic hyperplasia in the middle-aged and elderly males.

Zeng et al (2004) studied the curative effect of sporoderm-broken Lingzhi spores on menopause syndrome in elderly patients through data on their blood testosterone, SOD and MDA of erythrocytes, as well as psychological scores. In 138 cases of the male patients, who showed symptoms including fatigue, insomnia, contraction of blood vessels, spiritual and psychological symptoms and sexual dysfunction, their disease histories were 6 months to 2 years (averaging 12.3 months) and blood testosterone levels were lower than the normal level (140 mg/L). Age of the patients ranged from 55 to 76 years, averaging 66 years old. Sixty-one of them were single comprising 52.9% of the total. None of them suffered any serious cardiovascular, cerebrovascular, infectious diseases or malignant tumors. The patients' own evaluation scores on the partial androgen deficiency for middle-aged and elder men by SRS were higher than 16. The standard Zung Depression Scores were no less than 50. Those scores were used as guidelines for the diagnosis of meno-pause syndrome. Patients were randomly divided into 2 groups with 80 in the Treatment Group. Blood testosterone, SOD activity and MDA content of the fasting arterial blood were measured after patient's case history, Zung Depression and SRS scores were collected. Patients in the Treatment Group were given 600 mg Lingzhi spores capsules 3 times a day for 3 weeks, without any drugs for psychiatric treatment purpose. All patients were examined once a week for symptoms, as well as SRS and Zung Depression scores. Blood testosterone, SOD and MDA levels were determined 3 weeks after the beginning of Lingzhi administration. The Control Group of 58 patients was given a placebo.

After 3 weeks, patients in both groups showed different degrees of improvement on various menopausal symptoms. The SRS and Zung scores decreased significantly in the Treatment Group, while no significant changes were found in the Control Group. The total effective rate of the Treatment Group was 74.3%, significantly higher than that of the Control Group (i.e., 28.16%). The blood testosterone and SOD levels of the Treatment Group were significantly higher than those of the Control Group. The MDA levels of the Treatment Group were significantly lower than those of the Control Group (Table 11-5, 11-6 and 11-7). The results indicate that the sporoderm- broken Lingzhi spores has a therapeutic effect on male menopause syndrome.

Table 11-5 Number and percentage of cases with improvement on menopausal symptoms after treatment in Treatment and Control Groups

		malaise	anoxia	palpitation	forgetfulness	agitation	depression	impotence
Treatment	wk 1	46(57.5)	38(47.5)	26(32.5)	40(50)	22(27.5)	48(60)	56(70)
	wk 2	56(70)	50(62.5)	30(37.5)	42(52.5)	30(37.5)	56(70)	56(70)
	wk 3	70(85)*	56(70)*	30(37.5)*	42(52.5)*	30(37.5)*	66(82.5)*	64(80)
Control	wk 1	15(25)	11(20)	3(5)	7(12.5)	6(10)	11(20)	14(25)
	wk 2	20(35)	13(22.5)	4(7.5)	11(20)	9(15)	13(22.5)	17(30)
	wk 3	22(37.5)*	16(27.5)*	4(7.5)*	16(27.5)*	9(15)*	13(22.5)*	20(35)*

$\bar{x} \pm s$; *P <0.05, compared with sampling before treatment; percentage in parenthesis.

Table 11-6 Blood testosterone, SOD and MDA levels before and after treatment in Treatment and Control Groups

		Testosterone(mg/L)	SOD(U/g·Hb)	MDA(μmol/L)
Treatment	before treatment	131.5± 19.12	1068.3± 121.4	7.6± 0.8
	3 week afterward	253.72± 21.45*	1178.1± 132.6*	5.8± 0.6*
Control	before treatment	143.65± 20.31	1023.3± 101.6	7.1± 0.5
	3 week afterward	150.44± 17.46	1048.3± 112.4	7.3± 0.7

$\bar{x}±s$; $^*P<0.05$, compared with sampling before treatment

Table 11-7 Zung Depression and SRS scores before and after treatment in Treatment and Control Groups

		before treatment	1 week	2 week	3 week
Treatment	Zung score	54.36± 6.19	47.23± 6.93	42.71± 7.12	38.25± 6.56
	SRS score	21.26± 3.43	19.65± 3.14	17.96± 1.53	15.45± 3.42
Control	Zung score	53.12± 7.31	52.81± 7.15	50.32± 7.63	48.41± 6.75
	SRS score	22.12± 3.84	21.56± 6.23	21.13± 5.16	20.45± 4.33

All of the patients that used Lingzhi spores showed no significant adverse reactions. In the 2 patients, who suffered transient constipation, the problem disappeared during the course of the trial. There were no water or sodium retention, dysuria, liver and kidney function abnormalities observed during the trial.

Zeng, G.Q., Zong, W.D., Chung, Peter C.K. et al. Treatment of male menopause syndrome by Shell-broken *Ganoderma lucidum* spores. Guangzhou Medical College Journal 2004, 32 (1): 46-48)

Noguchi et al (2005) investigated the efficacy and safety of Lingzhi methanol extract on male patients with moderate bladder outlet obstruction (BOO). In their Phase I clinical trial, a randomized, double-blind, placebo-controlled experiment was conducted for 8 weeks. The International Prostate Symptom Score (I-PSS; Questionnaires 1-7) of the male volunteers (age 50) was not lower than 8, and the prostate specific antigen (PSA) was less than 4 ng/ml. When α -blockers or other drugs were used for treating the benign prostatic hyperplasia, they were stopped for 2 weeks prior to the trial. Volunteers were randomly divided into the placebo (12 patients), 0.6 mg methanol extract (12 patients), 6mg methanol extract (12 patients) and 60 mg methanol extract (14 patients) groups. They were administered placebo or various dosages of Lingzhi methanol extract once daily. Lingzhi's efficacy was determined by the changes in I-PSS, peak urine flow rate (Q_{max}), prostate size, residual urine estimated by ultrasonography, and blood tests, including PSA. No major adverse effects were observed during the entire course of the experiment. Compared to the placebo group, the I-PSS in the 6mg and 60mg dosage groups decreased significantly in the first 4 weeks and 8 weeks. There were no significant differences in Q_{max}, residual urine, prostate size or serum PSA between the 6 mg and 60 mg dosage groups. The results suggest that Lingzhi methanol extract clearly improved the symptoms on male patients with BOO. The authors recommended a dose of 6mg of the extract to be applied in their Phase II trial for patients with moderate BOO.

Noguchi, M., Kakuma, T., Tomiyasu, K. et al. Phase I study of a methanol extract of *Ganoderma lucidum*, and medicinal mushroom, in men with mild symptoms of bladder outlet obstruction. Urology, 2005, 66 (S 3A): 21)

In a recent article in the *Asian Journal of Andrology*, Lingzhi ethanol extract was reportedly to show significant effects on men with lower urinary tract symptoms (LUTS). Eighty-eight 49 years or older patients with mild to moderate LUTS were divided into treatment and control groups for the randomized, double-blind, placebo-controlled trial. The patients in the Treatment Group were administered 6 mg Lingzhi ethanol extract daily for 12 weeks, while the Control Group received the placebo. It was found that the I-PSS was significantly lower in the Treatment Group than the Control. However, no significant changes were found on other indicators, such as quality of sex life, Qmax, residual urine, prostate size, serum PSA and testosterone content.

Noguchi, M., Kakuma, T., Tomiyasu, K. et al. Randomized clinical trial of an ethanol extract of *Ganoderma lucidum* in men with lower urinary tract symptoms. Asian J Androl, 2008,10(5):777-85)

Health effects of Lingzhi on athletes

Zhang et al (1997) studied the effects of Lingzhi liquid on anti-fatigue, SOD, blood catalase (CAT) and LPO in athletes. Male athletes averaging 16.37 ± 1.7 years old were divided into treatment and control group with 13 subjects in each group. Those in the Treatment Group were administered 10 ml Lingzhi liquid twice a day for 30 days. Those in the Control Group were given placebo containing Coca-Cola to yield a similar appearance as Lingzhi liquid. Significantly longer exercise time with increasing load and higher work volume in the athletes were found after the treatment with Lingzhi liquid. This was also true when comparing the Treatment with the Control Group. After Lingzhi treatment, the hemoglobin content of the athletes increased from $14.43g\% \pm 0.49g\%$ to $15.73g\% \pm 0.54g\%$, while no significant change was found in the Control Group. The athlete's blood lactic acid content for the

Treatment Group was 9.32 ± 1.21 mmol/L 5 minutes after exercises. In 15 minutes, it decreased to 6.34 ± 1.31 mmol/L. There were significant differences between the two measurements. On the other hand, those for the Control Group were 9.88 ± 0.56 mmol/L and 8.47 ± 0.79 mmol/L in 5 and 15 minutes after exercises, respectively. There were no significant differences between them. In addition, Lingzhi liquid also significantly reduced the serum LPO, increased SOD, and enhanced hemoglobin and CAT activities. Consequently, by increasing hemoglobin content, accelerating blood lactic acid removal, enhancing SOD and CAT activities and inhibiting LPO formation, Lingzhi liquid improves endurance in exercise.

Zhang, A.M. et al. The *Ganoderma lucidum* liquid's effects on the anti-fatigue, SOD, CAT and LPO of blood in athletes. Chinese Journal of Sports Medicine, 1996, 6 (3): 19

Luo and Zhang (2006) studied the effects of Lingzhi capsules on CD35 of erythrocytes on athletes, who lived at 2500-meter altitude and trained at low altitude for 4 weeks. Sixteen soccer players from the Physical Education College at Beijing Sport University were recruited for the experiment. All participants were not residents in areas of high altitude, and had no pre-history of liver, kidney and endocrine diseases. Nor did they ever take any medications that could affect erythrocytes metabolism. They were randomly divided into treatment and control groups with 8 members in each group. All were subjected to the "lived high and trained low (LHTL)" regiment. Before living in the hypoxic room, the athletes in the Treatment group were administered 10 Lingzhi capsules (i.e., 0.25g per capsule consisting of 70% of Lingzhi fruiting body extract and 20% of Lingzhi spore powder) daily for 2 weeks. The Control Group had a placebo. The two groups lived in a hypoxic room, which had 15.4%

O_2 equivalent to 2500 meters altitude, for 10 hours per night. Twice a week, all were trained by means of the 72% maximum oxygen uptake bike training for 30 minutes in the hypoxic room. Concurrently, all were under the same training programs by the same coach 3 times a week. In the morning, venous blood samples were collected before Lingzhi administration and hypoxic exposure, as well as after 10 hours, 2 weeks, 3 weeks and 4 weeks living in the hypoxic room. With the fluorescent antibody response, the average fluorescence intensity and the rate of positive cells were recorded by means of flow cytometry. After 4 weeks, the erythrocytes CD35 expression of the Treatment Group increased by 7.9%, and that of the Control Group decreased by 12.8% ($P<0.05$). The red blood cell C3b receptor rosette rate of the Treatment Group increased by 45.9%, and that of the Control Group decreased by 49.0% ($P<0.05$). There were significant differences between the two groups. The erythrocytes immune complex rosette rate of the Treatment Group increased by 99.7% ($P <0.01$), and that of the Control Group increased by 19.5%. These results indicate that Lingzhi capsules could significantly increase erythrocytes CD35 expression, as well as improve erythrocytes secondary immunosuppressive response on athletes under the "LHTL" program. Luo, L. and Zhang, Y. Effects of Lingzhi capsules on the number and the activity of CD35 of erythrocytes in living high-training low athletes. Shanxi Sports Science and Technology, 2006, 26 (4) :38-41

The authors also reported, in another study, the effects of Lingzhi capsules on the number of the lymphocyte subtypes in soccer players during their 4 weeks "LHTL" program. Forty athletes were randomly and equally divided into Control Group (i.e., living under normal air pressure), LHTL Control Group, LHTL Treatment Group 1 and LHTL Treatment Group 2. Starting from 2 weeks before living in the hypoxic room, the Treatment Groups 1 and 2 were administered 2.5g and 5.0g Lingzhi capsules daily, respectively, for 6 weeks. The Control Groups were given a placebo during the same period of time. The ratio of CD4+/CD8+ was determined by using flow cytometry. It was found that, after 28 days of the experimentation, the CD4+/CD8+ ratios of the first 3 groups decreased significantly, but that of the Treatment Group 2 was higher than that of the LHTL Control and the Treatment Group 1. During the 6 weeks of the trial, there were no abnormalities found in blood biochemistry or the urine routine tests on the subjects. The results proved that significant reduction on the CD4+/CD8+ ratio could result from low-pressure, hypoxia or exercise-induced stress conditions, and that Lingzhi capsules could help alleviate the immunity lowering under such circumstances.

Zhang, Y., Lin, Z.B. and Wang, F. Effect of *Ganoderma Lucidum* Capsules on T-Lymphocyte Subsets in Soccer Players of Living High-Training Low. Br J Sports Med. 2008,42:519-522

Lingzhi has also been found effective in preventing high-altitude sickness. For example, Lingzhi tablet containing Lingzhi mycelium and Lingzhi Su-Xin tablet containing Lingzhi concentrated fermention liquid relieved the high altitude reaction on 469 cases. These products significantly reduced the incidence rate of acute mountain sickness (e.g., headaches, vomiting, etc.) at 4000-5000 m altitude. The effective rates of Lingzhi tablet and Lingzhi Su-Xin tablet were 98.6% and 97.5%, respectively.

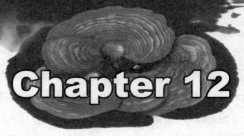

Chapter 12

Lingzhi Minimizes Poisoning Effect of Poisonous Mushrooms

Author's prompt: Poisoning from the poisonous mushrooms in the wild progresses rapidly and is oftentimes fatal. High mortality can result because there is no specific antidote available at present. Clinical practices indicate that incorporating Lingzhi with the conventional life-saving measures considerably reduces the death rate. Apparently, Lingzhi improves patient's chance of survival through its function in protecting the heart, liver and kidney. By reducing the toxic reactions and pathological changes on the affected organs, Lingzhi effectively minimizes the poisoning effect of the poisonous mushrooms.

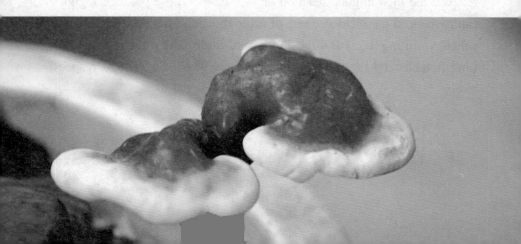

Mushroom poisoning

Eaten by mistake, poisonous mushrooms (fungi), such as Amanitaceae mushrooms (e.g., *Amanita verna* [(Bull. ex Fr) Pers.ex Vitt], *Amanita solitaria* [(Bull. ex Fr.) Karst], *Amanita pantherina* [(Dc. ex Fr.) Schrmm.]) and Russulaceae mushrooms (e.g., *Russula subnigricans* Hongo) can be deadly poisonous to human beings.

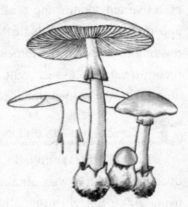

Of all the poisoning cases, 95% are caused by mistakenly eating Amanita mushrooms in the wild. The most lethal toxins in the mushrooms are amanitins. The toxins are bicyclic octapeptides. In the nature, there are 9 different amanitins, including α-amanitin. The amanitins are water soluble, chemically stable, as well as temperature, acid and alkali resistant. Upon ingestion, they are absorbed quickly through the digestive tract and transported to the liver. In the liver, it combines with RNA polymerase inhibiting mRNA formation, which results in necrosis of the liver cells followed by multi-organ failures due to the acute liver condition. Though slow-acting, amanitins give the following typical characteristics of poisoning: (a) apparent seasonality on occurrence in summer and autumn for mushroom harvest; (b) likely collective epidemiological incidences; (c) a higher than 60% mortality rate; (d) a typical clinical process with 3-6 hours incubation period, 24-48 hours acute gastroenteritis period, approximately a 24-48 hours latent period and a long visceral damage and recovery period, at which time the majority of death occurs; and (e) no specific antidote is available for the toxins at present.

As early as the 1970s, Lingzhi and Zizhi have been found to be an effective aid for treating mushroom poisoning. More recently, clinical and theoretical research further confirmed this application. Because mushroom poisoning is ferocious, severe and frequently fatal, it is not recommended to use Lingzhi alone, but is highly advisable to apply it along with the conventional clinical treatment for the poisoning.

Clinical reports on Lingzhi for Amanita mushroom poisoning

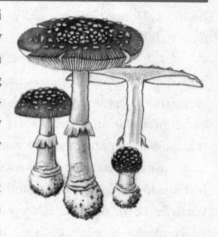

Li et al (2003) applied Lingzhi decoction, which was obtained by using 200 g Lingzhi fruiting body in water to simmer to 600 ml, in treating 25 cases of Amanita poisoning patients. The patients were given orally 200ml of the decoction 3 times a day for 7 days as a course of treatment. One to 2 courses of the treatment were applied for the trial. After the treatment, symptoms in all of the patients disappeared. Their serum total bilirubin (STB), bile acid (BA), alanine aminotransferase (ALT), aspartate aminotransferase (AST) and other indicators were back to or close to normal. At the time of admission, amanitin was detected in the blood of all patients. On the 3rd day, only a trace amount of the amanitin was found, and none on the 5th day after Lingzhi treatment.

Li, T.W., Xiao, Q.L. and Jin, Y.Q. A clinical report of treatment with lingzhi decoction on 25 cases of poisoning patients by amanita mushroom. Hunan Journal Of Traditional Chinese Medicine, 2003, 19(3): 17

Xiao et al (2003) also reported the therapeutic effect of Lingzhi decoction on Amanita mushroom poisoning. Twenty-three patients were randomly divided into treatment and control groups. Patients in the Control Group were given conventional medical care with penicillin and reduced glutathione. The Treatment Group was treated with addition of Lingzhi decoction (i.e., same as above). Patients in the Treatment Group were given orally 200 ml of the decoction 3 times a day for 7 days. Patients' STB, BA, ALT and AST increased initially in both groups. However, the indices peaked on the patients in the Treatment Group on the 3rd day of the treatment, and decreased significantly afterward. Whereas, these indices continued to rise on the patients in the Control Group. Comparing the indices of the 2 groups at the same time periods, significantly lower values were found in the Treatment than the Control Group. The results showed that Lingzhi decoction had a desirable therapeutic effect on treating the Amanita mushroom poisoning, and that a significantly reduced mortality rate was achieved among the patients with Lingzhi treatment.

Xiao, G.L., Liu, Y.F., Chen, Z.H. et al. A Clinical Study on the Therapeutic Effect of Lingzhi Decoction on the Poisoning Patients by Amanita Mushroom. Journal of TCM Univ. of Hunan, 2003, 43(1): 43-45

In another study, a 30% Zizhi decoction was administrated, along with the conventional medical care, to 11 patients of white Amanita mushroom [*Amanita verna* (Bull. ex Fr.) Pers. ex Vitt] poisoning at 50ml each time 3 times a day. All patients, except for one death, were cured after the treatment. Zizhi decoction has shown remarkable therapeutic results on Amanita poisoning when the central nerve system was damaged and the acute renal failure occurred. Zizhi continues to be used for treating other Amanita mushroom poisoning, such as *Amanita Pantherina* and *Amanita solitaria* (Bull. ex Fr.) Karst., with marked therapeutic efficacy as well.

Clinical reports on Lingzhi for *Russula subnigricans* poisoning

Russula subnigricans is another poisonous mushroom. It contains 4 different types of toxins, i.e., gastrointestinal, neurological, hemolytic and cytotoxic types, with fast action. Affected patients rapidly developed cellular damages in the liver and kidney. The renal necrosis, especially, can lead to death within 24 to 72 hours. *Russula subnigricans* is one of the most deadly poisonous mushrooms.

Xiao et al (2003) investigated the curative effect of Lingzhi decoction on patients of *Russula Subnigricans* poisoning. A group of 14 cases was treated, along with the conventional therapy, with Lingzhi decoction. The decoction was made with 100 g of Lingzhi fruiting body in water to simmer to 600 ml. 200ml of the decoction was administrated orally each time, except for unconscious patients, who had nasal feeding. The patients were given the decoction 3 times a day for 7 days as a course of treatment. According to a patient's conditions, 1–2 courses of the treatment were used. Another group of 11 patients, who were patients of the previous year, was used for comparison purpose. These patients received only the conventional treatment, such as oxygen and transfusion.

The parameters used for the comparison included the urine N-acetyl-D-glucosaminidase (NAG), red blood cell and protein in urine (which reflects kidney injury), ALT (which reflects liver injury) and AST (which reflects heart injury). The results pointed out that after Lingzhi treatment, a patient's condition quickly improved with no fatality. On the other hand, among the patients treated with only the conventional means, 3 died in 24 hours, 2 in 24–48 hours and 3 in 48–72 hours, i.e., a total of 8 deaths while in hospital. For the most of the patients, who received Lingzhi decoction, their red blood cells in urine completely disappeared after 24 hours of the treatment. Their urine protein was also significantly reduced, while NAG, ALT and AST rose to a peak in 3 days followed by a gradual decline. In contrast, those with the above mentioned parameters for patients in the group for comparison increased continuously. And, they were significantly higher than those of the group being treated with Lingzhi decoction. The results indicate that Lingzhi decoction is therapeutically effective in treating *Russula Subnigricans* poisoning, and that it can significantly reduce the mortality rate resulting from the poisoning.

Xiao, G.L., Liu, Y. and Chen, Z.H. Clinical observation on treatment of *Russula subnigricans* Poisoning Patients by Lingzhi decoction. Chinese Journal of Integrated Traditional Western Medicine, 2003, 23 (4); 278-280

Mechanism of therapeutic efficacy of Lingzhi on mushroom poisoning

Pharmacological studies on the effect of Lingzhi on mushroom poisoning not only confirmed the clinical findings, but also began to elucidate the mechanism associated with the therapeutic efficacy. In rabbits poisoned by the Amanita mushrooms, Lingzhi decoction significantly retarded the increasing activities of AST, lactate dehydrogenese (LDH), α-hydroxybutyric acid, creatine kinase (CK) and creatine kinase isoenzyme (CK-MB). At the same time, it significantly reduced the histopathological changes of myocardial injury in the poisoned rabbits. In addition, while improving the animal's liver functions, Lingzhi also

significantly increased the RNA polymerase activity, which was ill affected by the toxin. This latter function might play an important role in
the mechanism of Lingzhi's protective effect on the liver damage in poisoned rabbits.

Furthermore, Lingzhi decoction was found to significantly improve
the renal function and reduce the histopathological poisoning in the
kidney of the acute *Russula subnigricans* poisoned rats.

The reason that Lingzhi decoction has a detoxification effect on
Amanita mushroom poisoning might relate to its ability in minimizing
damages on the heart, liver and kidney induced by the toxins. By preventing multiple organ failures, Lingzhi helps in a patient's battle for
survival.

Yang, Y., Xiao, G.L ., Yang, N. et al. Protective effects of *Ganoderma
lucidum* on heart injury induced by Amanita poisoning in rabbits. Central South Pharmacy, 2006, 4(3): 171-174

Xiao, G., Xiong, J., Luo, C.D. et al. Protective efficacy of Lingzhi decoction on acute renal injury caused by *Russula subnigr*icans in rats. Journal
40 of TCM Univ. of Hunan, 2007, 27(5):40-43

Xiao, Q.L., Yang, N., Zhang, C.H. et al. Mechanism and protective effect
of glossy ganoderma decoction on the activities of RNA polymerase in
hepatocyte of rabbits with Amanita mushroom poisoning. J Cent South
Univ (M ed Sci), 2007,32(4): 637-640

Chapter 13

Lingzhi for Treatment of Other Diseases

Author's prompt: *G. capense* injection has been used for treatment of nephrotic syndrome, alopecia areata and localized scleroderma. Lingzhi spore injection has shown an effect on treatment of multiple sclerosis and myotonia atrophica. In addition, Lingzhi, in combination with anti-retroviral drugs, has been found to improve health conditions in AIDS patients.

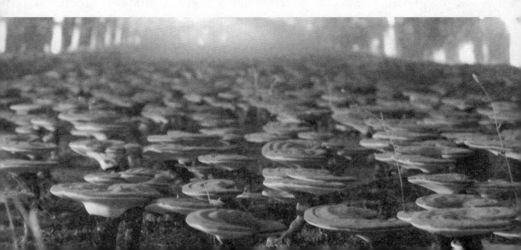

Preliminary studies showed that Lingzhi could be used in treating several diseases other than those described in the previous chapters. They are discussed as follows.

 For nephrotic syndrome

Li et al (2003) reported the therapeutic effect of *G. capense* injection on 42 patients with nephrotic syndrome. From 1999 to 2001, 82 hospitalized nephrotic patients, 57 male and 25 female at 12-60 years old (averaging 27.1 ± 7), were selected for the study. All patients had been diagnosed with nephrotic syndrome according to the guidelines of the Chinese Medical Association and those of WHO established in 1982. The guidelines include: (a) severe proteinuria $\geq 315g/24h$, and (b) hypoproteinemia: total protein < 60 g/L and serum albumin $< 30g/L$, with or without edema and hyperlipidemia. Among the patients, 77 had the primary nephrotic syndrome, 4 lupus nephropathy and 1 hepatitis B-related nephropathy. None of them had been treated for the diseases before the trial. They either had no, or only moderate, renal dysfunction. Some patients had different degrees of anemia, and 3 cases were accompanied by venous thrombosis of the lower extremity and 24 with infections. These 82 patients were randomly divided into observation and control groups. There were no significant differences in gender, age or renal function on the patients between the 2 groups. In the Observation Group of 42 patients, 28 were male and 14 female between the age 12 and 59 (averaging 28.7 ± 5 years old). They included 39 cases of primary nephrotic syndrome, 2 lupus nephropathy and 1 hepatitis B-related nephropathy. Hormones, along with 2 ampoules of the *G. capense* injection (i.e., 2 ml/ampoule containing 500 mg *G. capense* extract in each ampoule), received intramuscular injections twice every day for 84 days.

In the Control Group, the 40 patients, 29 males and 11 females with ages between 14 and 60 (averaging 25.8±7 years old), consisted of 38 with primary nephrotic syndrome and 2 with lupus nephropathy. The standard hormone treatment of a daily injection of prednisone at the dosage rate of 1–115 mg/kg was applied for all participating patients. In addition, for expansion of blood volume and anticoagulation, both groups were dosed with 250–500 ml of a low molecular weight dextran and 160 mg of ligustrazine by intravenous drip for 14–21 days. And, for electrolyte modulation and infection control, symptomatic treatments were given to patients when needed.

Clinical observations, such as dizziness, acratia, edema, chest distress, palpitation, dyspnea, abdominal distension, anorexia, blood pressure and body weight, on the patients were recorded. Laboratory tests were also performed. They included: (a) routine blood and urine tests, qualitative and quantitative urine protein tests (once a week), (b) urine protein electrophoresis, serum albumin, cholesterol, triglycerides, creatinine, immunoglobulin, complement and T cell subsets (once a month), and (c) renal biopsies under microscope, electron microscope and immuno-fluoroscope.

Classifications of the clinical efficacy included: cure, excellent, effective and failed. "Cure" was defined as elimination of symptoms, physical signs and complications; "excellent" was elimination of most symptoms; "effective" was amelioration of symptoms and physical signs; and, "failed" showed no apparent changes.

In the Observation Group, 22 cases of "cure" (i.e., 52.4% of the total), 13 of "excellent" (i.e., 30.9%), 5 of "effective" (i.e., 11.9%) and 2 of "failed" (i.e., 4.8%) were found. The total effective rate was 95.2%, which was significantly higher than that in the Control Group (i.e.,

53.2%) (P <0. 05).

The urine protein electrophoresis showed 17 cases of selective proteinuria (i.e., 43.3%) and 25 non-selective proteinuria (59.5%) in the Observation Group prior to the trial. After the treatment, 7 transformed from the non-selective to the selective proteinuria (i.e., 28.0%). On the other hand, in the Control Group, there were 19 cases of selective proteinuria (i.e., 47.5%) and 21 non-proteinuria (i.e., 52.5%) prior to the trial, and only 4 (i.e., 19.0%) transformed after the treatment. The urinary protein recovery time in the Observation Group showed 9 cases of recovery in 28 days (i.e., 21.4%), 20 cases in 42 days (i.e., 47.3%) and 13 cases in 56 days (i.e., 39.2%), with the peak occurring in 4-6 weeks. No recurrence was found. In contrast, in the Control Group, 5 cases of recovery in 42 days (i.e., 12.5% recovery rate) were found with 3 recurrences, i.e., at a recurrence rate of 60%, in the course of medication. There were 16 cases of recovery in 56 days (i.e., 40.0% recovery rate) with 7 recurrences (at a recurrence rate of 43.8%), and 24 cases of recovery in 84 days (i.e., 60% recovery rate) with 3 recurrences after six months (at a recurrence rate of 12.5%). The urinary protein recovery time for the Observation Group was 4 weeks shorter than the Control Group. There were no cases of recurrence in the Observation Group, whereas the Control Group had 13 cases, i.e., a recurrence rate of 32.5%. Patients, who had hyperlipemia or mild renal damage, improved significantly after the treatment. Other indicators, such as Hb, immunoglobulin IgG, IgA, IgM, complement C3, T-lymphocyte subsets CD3, CD4, CD8 and CD4/CD8 were all enhanced by varying degrees.

Sixteen renal biopsies were conducted. The microscopy displayed infiltration of inflammatory cells in the renal interstitium, hyperplasia of fibrous connective tissue, regional focal glassy changes, degeneration, cast and atrophy in tubular. After 84 days treatment with *G. capense*, renal glomerular, tubular and interstitial lesions were reduced significantly. The electron microscopy showed a normal foot process structure, a clear three-tier structure of the basement membrane and no subepithelial electron-dense deposits after the treatment. Before the treatment, no change was found in the immunofluorescence of 4 cases of minor lesions. But, granular or linear type of IgG, C3 strong positive fluorescent staining in glomerular capillary wall were seen in 11 cases, especially in 3 systemic lupus erythematosus (SLE) cases. After 84 days of the treatment, one case turned into the membranous type, one into the membranous proliferative type, and the IgG, C3 fluorescence changed from positive to mild.

Nephrotic syndrome is a very common chronic kidney disease with multiple causes and various pathohistological changes. It is chronic in nature with high recurrence rates and diverse complications. Thus, it is challenging to find a treatment that can shorten the duration of the disease, increase the efficacy, reduce the recurrence rate and side effects, as well as prevent complications. To date, the main treatment objectives remain to be the reducing urinary protein excretion, increasing plasma proteins, especially albumin, shortening the disease duration to prevent complications, and protecting renal function. It is encouraging to see the synergistic effect demonstrated when TCM is applied in combination with conventional medications. The abovementioned study showed the adjuvant effect of *G. capense* in treating nephrotic patients with hormone. The significantly improved overall effective rate, shortened disease duration, reduced recurrence rate, decreased side effects, reversed and/or enhanced renal function, and minimized pathological damage to the kidney tissue were all a result of this promising medical approach.

Li, Y.Y., Ma, Y.R. and Liu, J. Clinical and experimental study of *Ganoderma capense* combined with hormone injection on treatment of nephrotic syndrome. Sichuan Medical Journal, 2003, 23(5):441-443

 ## For multiple sclerosis and myotonia atrophica

The treatment applying a Lingzhi preparation (i.e., once a day intramuscular injection of 400 mg Lingzhi spores) on 5 cases of multiple sclerosis by the Neurology Division at Beijing Friendship Hospital, and 10 cases of myotonia atrophica by H.T. Fu showed a certain improvements on the patients' symptoms. Since there is still no effective therapy available for treating multiple sclerosis or myotonia atrophica, Lingzhi's effects in relieving symptoms and strengthening muscles are noteworthy, nonetheless. It could potentially provide benefits in the treatment for such debilitating ailments.

 ## For scleroderma

Scleroderma is a disease of the connective tissues. The cause(s) of the disease remain unclear, and there is no satisfactory therapy available currently. Li et al (2000) reported a clinical observation of using *G. capense* injection for local scleroderma. Fifty-two patients with confirmed scleroderma by biopsy and the diagnostic criteria recommended by the American College of Rheumatology participated in the study. These were patients with a history of the disease for 3 months to 7 years (averaging 36.8±17.5 months), and of 4 males and 48 females between the ages of 7–54 years old. Their major invasion sites were on the face, lower limbs and body, and rarely involved the upper limbs. A few patients had multiple affected sites. The apparent symptoms shown on the sites included skin sclerosis, atrophy, burnish, pigmentation, trichomadesis, as well as localized dermatrophia and joint dysfunction in some patients. In addition to routine tests, antinuclear antibody (ANA), erythrocyte sedimentation rate (ESR), immunocomplex, immunoglobulin (i.e., IgG, IgA and IgM) and complement C3 and C4 were also measured. There were 5 cases of immunocomplex positive, 9 ESR elevation, 7 IgG increase and 3 IgM increase. 2ml/ampoule, which contained 0.5 g *G. capense* extract, were used for local injection of 2-4ml per site, once or twice a week for treatment. In the cases, where multiple sites were found, 2 sites were treated each time and no more than 8ml were applied totally each time. Continuous treatment of 12 weeks was a cycle. Among the 52 patients, the number of the treatment cycles varied from 1 to 3, averaging a total of 32.4 injections per site. The results were as follows: (a) 14 cases of short term cure (i.e., 26.9% of total) manifested by "the hardened, shrunk skin becoming normal, skin of the lesions returning to normal or almost normal color, joint dysfunction disappearing and hair growing;" (b) 29 cases of excellent (i.e., 55.8%) manifested by "more than 60% improvement on skin sclerosis, atrophy, pigmentation and dysfunction;" and (c) 9 cases of effective (i.e., 17.3%) manifested by "more than 20% improvement on skin sclerosis, atrophy, pigmentation and dysfunction". A total of 87 lesion sites were treated, with 18 sites resulted in short term cure (i.e., 20.7%), 56 in excellent (i.e., 64.4%) and 13 in effective classification (i.e., 14.9%). The biopsy examination showed that the thickened skin had attenuated, keratinization reduced, perivascular infiltration of inflammatory cells disappeared, collagen fibers thinned, and collagenoblast decreased. During the injection treatment, 4 patients had local skin rash and mild itching, which disappeared within 24 hours. 2 patients complained of dizziness and palpitations, and were relieved upon dose reduction. No other adverse reactions were reported.

Li, S.Z. et al Clinical observations of *Ganoderma capense* injection in the treatment of 52 cases of local scleroderma. Chinese Journal of Integrated Traditional and Western Medicine, 2000, 20:148)

Pharmacological studies have shown that extracts of Lingzhi fruiting body, mycelium and spores can protect chemical and immune injury on the muscles of the mice, reduce the elevation of serum aldolase induced by herbicide 2,4-dichlorophenoxyacetic acid in mice, and alleviate myotonia symptoms. Intraperitoneal injection of the water extract of Lingzhi spores significantly decreased the elevated serum phosphocreatine kinase (SCPK) and the depressed muscle phosphocreatine kinase (MCPK) activities in the muscles of the mice with immune injury. Meanwhile, pathological changes of muscle cell degeneration and necrosis were also relieved. Further study suggested that Lingzhi's ability to inhibit lipid peroxidation in muscle cell membrane caused by oxygen free radicals might contribute to muscle injury protection in mice. It could be one of the mechanisms that yielded the curative effect of Lingzhi on a certain muscular diseases.

 ## For alopecia areata

Cao et al (1986) reported the effect of *G. capense* preparations on 232 cases of alopecia areata at 4 hospitals. The patients, 157 male and 75 female, included 204 alopecia areata and 28 alopecia totalis cases. They were given either daily intramuscular injection of 2 ampoules of *G. capense* preparation or 3 times daily oral administration of 4 *G. capense* tablets for 2-4 months. Either injection ampoules or oral tablets were used in the treatment. The two methods were applied alternately on occasion as well. Clinical efficacy was judged and classified as: "cure", which was when full hair re-growth with a few gray hairs was shown; "excellent", when 60% or more partial hair re-growth was shown; "improved", when 20% or more hair re-growth was shown; and "failed", when no hair growth was observed.

After the treatment, there were 70 cases that fell into the "cure" category (i.e., 30.17% of the total), 51 in the "excellent" (i.e., 21.98%), 62 in the "improved" (i.e., 26.72%), and 49 in the "failed" category (i.e., 21.12%). The total number of effective cases was 183 (i.e., 78.88%). With the treatment, most of the patients said their appetite and sleep quality improved, headache and dizziness disappeared, and body weight and physical strength increased.

Cao, R.L., Wang, G.Z., Xie, J.H. et al. Clinical report of *Ganoderma capense* in treatment of alopecia areata. Journal of the Second Beijing Medical University, 1986, 7(3):217-218

For chloasma

Zhang et al (2002) studied the therapeutic effect of Lingzhi water extract/L-cysteine cream on chloasma. The cream was made with 20.0g of the Lingzhi water extract, 1.0g L-cysteine, 6.0g stearic acid, 3.0g cetyl alcohol, 3.0g monoglyceride, 12.0g white oil, 2.0g vaseline, 5.0g glycerol, 1.0g triethanolamine, 0.1g ethyl hydroxybenzoate and the balance of purified water to a total weight of 100.0 g. Separately heat the water phase (including glycerol, triethanolamine, ethyl hydroxybenzoate and the purified water) and the oil phase (including stearic acid, cetyl alcohol, monoglyceride and the white oil) to 80℃. Add the Lingzhi water extract to the water phase and mix well. Pour the water phase mixture slowly into the oil phase with stirring in one direction till the temperature drops to below 50 ℃. Add the cysteine solution and appropriate amount of essence for fragrance, and continue stirring until a milky white cream was obtained.

Randomly divided 121 chloasma outpatients that included 5 males and 116 females at the age of 24−55 years old into a treatment group of 61 and a control group of 60 patients. The patients had the disease for 1 month to 10 years, but were never treated medically. The two groups were comparable with respect to gender, age, as well as mottle area and distribution. Pregnant women, patients, who were taking oral contraceptives or had diseases that could lead to chloasma, and minors were all excluded from the study. For the Treatment Group, the compounded Lingzhi cream was applied, while the Control Group hydroquinone cream (containing mainly 2% hydroquinone) was given. The cream was uniformly smeared on the face followed by massaging on the mottled area for a few minutes. The treatment was done twice a day for 3 months. No other similar drugs or cosmetic products were allowed during the entire treatment period. The efficacy criteria included "cure" for equal or greater than 90% of the pigmented area dissipated and normal color returned; "excellent" for more than 60% of the pigmented area dissipated and the skin color lightened; "improved" for more than 30% of the pigmented area dissipated and the skin color greatly lightened; and, "failed" for less or equal to 30% of the pigmented area dissipated and without visible change on the skin color. The total effective rate was the sum of the rates of "cure" plus "excellent."

After the treatment, the total effective rate found in the Treatment Group was 82.0%, which is significantly higher than that in the Control group, i.e., 65.0%. A 6-month follow-up visit with the patients revealed a lost and a recurrence case in the Treatment Group, and one recurrence in the Control Group. The adverse reactions among the patients included

2 cases of skin rash, 2 cases of itching in the Treatment Group, and 2 cases of skin rash, 3 cases of itching, 2 cases of erythema and a case of swelling in the Control Group. The patient, who had swollen patches, received appropriate treatment and later withdrew from the project. Those remaining were not given any particular treatment as the side effects disappeared with the continued Lingzhi cream treatment.

Both Lingzhi water extract and L-cysteine are anti-oxidants with free radical scavenging ability. L-cysteine has an additional inhibitive effect on dopa and tyrosinase. Therefore, it can reduce melanocyte enzyme activity resulting in mottle-dissipation and skin-whitening. Consequently, by combining the two agents, the cream was effective in removing mottled skin, inhibiting dermatitis and delaying skin aging.

Zhang, A.J., Ge, W.Y., Wang, Y.T. et al. Preparation and effect of compound *Ganoderma lucidum* cream in the treatment of chloasma. The Chinese Journal of Dermatovenereology, 2002, 16(4):235-236

 ## For the acquired immune deficiency syndrome (AIDS)

In vitro studies showed that extracts of Lingzhi fruiting body and spores inhibited the reverse transcriptase and protease activities of the human immunodeficiency virus (HIV). Along with its immunoregulatory activities, Lingzhi was thus believed to have the potential for AIDS treatment.

In recent years, scientists have attempted to use Lingzhi for treating AIDS. For instance, in 2005, Mshigeni et al presented the results of their preliminary study on Lingzhi extract as an adjuvant agent for HIV/AIDS treatment. In that study, 46 HIV/AIDS patients were divided into two groups. One of the groups with 24 patients received anti-retroviral (ARV) drug therapy. The other group had ARV, along with Lingzhi extract.

The health promoting effects of Lingzhi extract in the HIV/AIDS patients observed in the study included the weight-gain, as well as elevations in the CD4 cell and hemoglobin counts. Consequently, a synergistic, or adjuvant, effect might exist when Lingzhi and ARV were used in combination for treating HIV/AIDS.

Mshigeni, K.E., Mtango, D., Massele, A. et al. Intriguing biological treasures more precious than gold: The case of tuberous truffles, and immunomodulating *Ganoderma* mushrooms with potential for HIV /AIDS treatment. Discovery and Innovation, 2005, 17:105-109

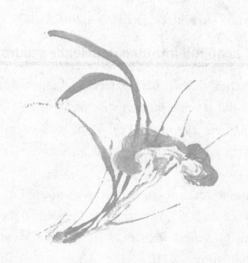

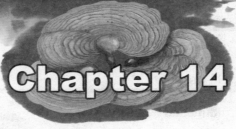

Chapter 14

Recommendations in Choosing and Using Lingzhi Products

Author's prompt: There is a variety of Lingzhi products on the market. Lingzhi can be artificially cultivated or harvested from the wild. Its products may be in the crude forms, such as fruiting body slices and spore powder. There are also products formulated for medicinal, dietary supplement and cosmetic applications. Variations in quality and efficacy, as well as information on appropriate applications are of interest to the consumers. Recommendations in this regards are summarized so that Lingzhi's therapeutic effect and health functions can be maximized and safety assured.

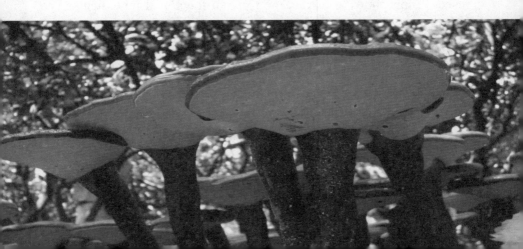

Lingzhi products

Many rudimentary Lingzhi products, such as fruiting body slices or
pieces and spore powder, are available
on the market. They may be cheaper,
but not always better, than further processed items. Their quality should be
carefully scrutinized before purchasing.
For example, the fruiting body is lower

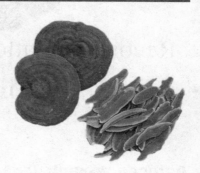

in its potency after than before spore-ejection. The spores collected are
called "powder" because their powdery appearance of them. They are
not a "processed" product. Spore powder may be intentionally or by
nature to include adulterants. As a result, the product would be inferior
in quality. Unfortunately, it is rather difficult to distinguish the good
from the bad with the naked eye. Lingzhi slices or spore powder are
commonly simmered in water to get decoction before use. In cooking
them, it is best to cut the fruiting body slices into small pieces to facilitate
the extraction. After the initial decoction is collected, the pulp can be
used 3 more times to extract the residual functional ingredients. The
final cooked residue can still be marinated in a 50% alcoholic content
liquor to obtain the alcohol-soluble components left behind. In 15 to
20 days, the alcohol-solubles will turn the liquor reddish brown. This
tonic alcoholic beverage, as well as the water decoction, can be taken
twice daily at the rate of 6–12g (as the raw material weight) per day. For
the spore powder, the recommended daily dosage is 5g by taking it twice
a day.

Medicinal products: Medicines can be made from the fruiting

body, mycelium or spores of Lingzhi, as they all contain active components in varying amounts. The products can be in the form of tablets, capsules or instant powder or granules. In general, these types of products are processed by extraction, encapsulation and/or formulation. As a result, they are normally purer and better in quality, as well as easier for the body to absorb and utilize than the raw materials. Nonetheless, in purchasing these products, the information on the product, including ingredients, net weight, claims, manufacturer, license and permit numbers from the authorities and date code should be carefully examined. Before taking the product, the instructions that accompany the product on applications, dosage, possible side effects, etc. should be read and understood thoroughly, and followed faithfully.

Health food products: Health food is also known as functional or nutraceutical food. In the U.S., dietary supplements can also be considered in the same category. Despite difference in the names, these products are made from raw materials with formulation and precautions on usage similar to those for medicines. By definition, drugs are used for and proven effective in curing specific diseases, whereas a health food or dietary supplement product is limited to its claim and efficacy for health benefits only.

 ## Quality of Lingzhi products

In general, Lingzhi refers to the fruiting body of *G. lucidum*, a member of the big family of *Ganoderma* genus. Lingzhi can be harvested either from the wild or cultivation farms.

At present, 3 forms of the fruiting body products are most commonly available on the market, i.e., the whole body, cut pieces and ground powder. It is rather difficult to judge the quality of the cut or ground products by the naked eye. A microscope or chemical analysis needs to be used for this purpose. On the raw whole fruiting body, color, thickness and weight can offer clues to its quality. The desirable fruiting body of a Lingzhi plant grown on a log has a round or kidney shape, and its stem is short and the cap thick. On the bottom of the cap, where the tubular channels can be seen with a magnifier, the color should be light or golden yellow to be of the highest quality. If the color is white, the fruiting body is considered to be of secondary quality. If the color has turned grayish white, the fruiting body's quality is the least desirable. At that stage, the plant has already completed its spore ejection, leaving it with the least amount of the active ingredients in the fruiting body.

 ## Misconception on quality of wild Lingzhi

Lingzhi is scarcely found in the wild nowadays. Some may believe that the wild Lingzhi is of premium quality. In fact, though scarce, Lingzhi picked in the wild is not necessarily superior to its cultivated counterpart. First of all, more than 70 different species of wild Lingzhi found in China have been identified as belonging to the *Ganoderma* genus (see chapter 3). The pharmacological and toxicological properties of most of these species are not known. Consequently, only three kinds of ganoderma are listed as drugs in the *Chinese Pharmacopoeia*. Many polypore fungi commonly grow along side Lingzhi in the wild. It is difficult to distinguish between them and Lingzhi. Yet, ingestion of these polypore fungi can cause harm to human beings. Secondly, there is no evidence to support the claim of a superior pharmalogical effect existing in the wild Lingzhi. Lastly, Lingzhi plants in the wild are more susceptible to insect infestation and mold infection than they are under an artificially controlled environment. Lingzhi grown under proper cultivation conditions should be adequate for either medicinal or health purposes.

Some Lingzhi products stress their wild and natural origins. It is desirable to be pure and natural, but those so-called "wild" merchandise pose risks, as far as quality and safety are concerned. Drugs and health foods demand the highest possible quality and safety, which can only be achieved through stringently monitoring and control from raw material to the finished products. When a manufacturer collects wild Lingzhi from numerous and largely unknown sources, the quality of the fruiting body would make it impossible to adhere to any respectable standards. As expected, the quality of the products made from such raw materials would not be possible to track and maintain at a high and consistent level.

 ## Ways to distinguish good from bad Lingzhi products

☆   Lingzhi products without formal approval for sale by the State Food and Drug Administration (SFDA) are not reliable, nor safe to use. Therefore, it is prudent to make certain that a product bears the approval number(s) on the package. In China, an herbal product should show "Approval Number: State Drug Approval Z×××××××", and for a health food product, an "Approval Number: State Food Approval G×××××××". (Incidentally, the first 4 digits of these numbers refer to the year when the approval was granted by the authority.)

☆   Those Lingzhi products, which are not extracted from the raw materials, may be simply ground up from the fruiting body and/or mycelium into powder and filled in gel capsules. The possible existence of adulterants, such as fibers and debris, will reduce the potential efficacy of the Lingzhi products.

☆   Some so-called "whole plant" Lingzhi products are made of mixtures of fruiting body extract and spores. They are not necessarily of premium quality. In fact, the best quality Lingzhi fruiting body products are made of fruiting bodies at the stage, when the light-yellowish growing line on the edge of the cap has just disappeared, before the spores are ejected. At this stage, the fruiting body contains the peak amount of all active components.

☆   If the raw materials have been contaminated with heavy metals (e.g., arsenic, mercury and lead) and/or pesticides, the resultant Lingzhi products can invariably carry those harmful elements that can be detrimental to our health.

☆   Lingzhi teas or drinks are convenient to use, but often formulated with ingredients, such as sugar and starch. They are, thus, not only diluted, as far as the Lingzhi content is concerned, but also undesirable for the elderly and/or diabetic patients.

☆   Some Lingzhi products claim to have high germanium and/or selenium contents. However, germanium is neither an essential mineral for human health, nor is it considered an active component for Lingzhi. And, there is no scientific evidence that supports any additional therapeutic effect of germanium in Lingzhi. As for selenium, although it is a necessary trace element for humans, its overdose can cause harm. For those who do not have a selenium deficiency, there is no need for such a supplement. Regardless, it has never been proven that Lingzhi enriched with selenium had an improved efficacy.

☆   There were products advertised as "Five Color Lingzhi" meaning that they were produced using Lingzhi of 5 different colors, as indicated in the ancient TCM literature. As discussed in Chapter 2, the yellow and white Lingzhi are not even considered *G. lucidum.*

☆　　　Lingzhi spores have two layers of cell walls. The spore oil and other active ingredients enclosed inside these cell walls cannot be efficiently released and absorbed by the body unless the cell walls are broken. Thus, intact spores packed directly in capsules have been found in feces.

☆　　　When the spore's cell walls are broken, spore oil and other active ingredients can leach out easily and be readily utilized by the body. The bio-availability of the spore product can thus be greatly enhanced. Therefore, the percentage of the broken spores in a spore product is a critical factor in evaluating its quality. A report published by the Customer Committee of Hong Kong indicated that of 16 commercial Lingzhi products that they examined, only 8 showed greater than 90% cell wall breakage rates. More shockingly, they found 2 of the sampled products had a rate less than 20%, and one merely 5%! Variation in quality of the spore products on the market is a stark reality and alarming. On the other hand, the spore oil contains a high amount of unsaturated fatty acids, cell wall breakage allows its full exposure to air that can accelerate oil oxidation or rancidity. Hence, the packaging and storage for the spore oil products must take these factors into consideration.

☆　　　The lipids, unsaturated fatty acids and triterpenes in the spore oil are susceptible to oxidization and degradation when exposed to air. To protect them, minimizing air infiltration by using appropriate capsules and packaging material, preventing oxidation by employing anti-oxidant agents, such as Vitamin E, and avoiding high temperature exposures are highly recommended. Should any rancid, off flavor be detected in a product, it should be discarded.

 Polysaccharide content in Lingzhi products

Polysaccharides are important active components in Lingzhi. Its content is an essential criterion for judging the quality of the raw material as well as the finished products. The 2005 edition of the *Chinese Pharmacopoeias Part I* sets a standard for the polysaccharide content, as anhydrous dextrose, in dried Lingzhi fruiting body to be no less than 0.5%.

In manufacturing spray-dried Lingzhi powdered products, additives, such as dextrin, are frequently applied. To form tablets or fill capsules, starches are also commonly added to facilitate the operation. In making instant powder or granules, again, starch or dextrin is used. Besides, starch is a bulking agent where highly concentrated Lingzhi or drug ingredients need to be diluted to meet dosage requirements. Therefore, using dextrose (AKA glucose) as an index in analysis to determine the polysaccharide content in Lingzhi cannot truly reflect the product quality. Worse yet, such a method encourages fraudulent acts. The misleading information has caused much confusion as a result.

To remedy the problem, attempts have been made to use alternative index or indices, such as the purified peptidoglycan in *G. lucidum*, rather than dextrose. New standards and analytical methods to identify Lingzhi product quality are also in the making in China. Despite the difficulties, establishment of evaluation criteria and an acceptable methodology is urgently needed in order to protect the consumer interest, as well as for progress in the industry and promotion of the mysteriously wonderful Lingzhi for the benefit of human health.

 ## Side effects or "vertigo-like therapeutic"?

It has been rare to find side effects in clinical applications of Lingzhi. Only occasionally, patients were found to suffer gastrointestinal discomfort, abdominal distention, diarrhea, constipation, dry mouth, dry pharynx or lip blistering. These side effects were either light in nature, or they gradually disappeared upon continuous administration of Lingzhi. Stopping the use was not seen as necessary. In clinical trials, Lingzhi has not shown any significant adverse effects on the heart, liver, kidney or other vital organs. This is consistent with what was recorded in TCM literature indicating that Lingzhi1was not toxic, even with long-term use.

To divert the consumer's attention to the occasional and slight side effects of Lingzhi, some tried to theorize the non-toxicity of Lingzhi as "vertigo-like therapeutic" reactions on the patients. They would further suggest that those reactions were inevitable for the in vivo detoxification. Their attempt to explain Lingzhi's function is totally unnecessary. Any drug can, more or less, produce side effects. Lingzhi is no exception.

 ## Misdiagnosis of Lingzhi spores as parasite eggs

More than a dozen cases of misdiagnosing Lingzhi spores as parasite eggs in the intestine were reported. When feces were examined under a microscope, similarities between the spores and the parasite eggs caused erroneous diagnosis. Under a microscope, the spores are light brown in color and shaped like watermelon seeds with a size close to the lymphocyte. Lingzhi spore has two thick layers of cell walls. One end of the spore is sharper than the other and has no cap-like structure. The other end is blunt and round with no miliary spine or miracidium inside. The appearance of a spore is much like the eggs of *Distoma hepaticum* and *Distoma japonicum*. Incorrect diagnosis can lead to wrong treatment. To avoid the mistake, it is recommended that the patients be asked whether they use Lingzhi or Lingzhi spore products. After patients stop taking Lingzhi, the "egg-shaped" substances should disappear, and re-appear when Lingzhi is administered again. By smearing a sample of the Lingzhi product with a drop of saline solution on the slide for observation under a microscope to compare with the fecal sample, it should become apparent whether the patient contracted a parasitic disease or not. Naturally, the patient ought to inform the physician of the use of Lingzhi product in advance to avoid confusion on the examination.

Presence of the spores in feces suggests that Lingzhi spores can be difficult to be digested by humans. Consequently, breaking the spore cell wall prior to ingestion may improve the bio-availability and maximize the efficacy of the spore products.

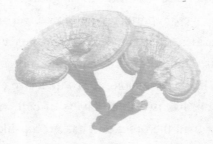

Chapter 15

Processing Technology for Lingzhi Products

Author's prompt: A variety of Lingzhi products can be made from its fruiting body, mycelium or spores. The traditional herbal extraction to produce decoctions, syrups and pastes, as well as the solvent and supercritical fluid extraction methods to yield concentrated and/or isolated compounds for oral applications or injection ampoules have all been applied to obtain some of the further processed products seen on the market today. More recently, the submerged fermentation with selected Lingzhi strains have been used to grow and collect active compounds directly from the liquid culture medium, rather than logs or bags with formulated dry ingredients. These materials can be either pressed to form tablets, filled in capsules, pouched as instant mixes, sterilized as injection ampoules, or bottled for oral administration.

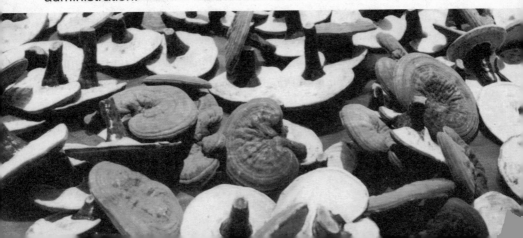

There is a wide variety of Lingzhi preparations that can be found on the market nowadays. They may come in the form of tablets, hard or soft-gel capsules, instant mixes, syrups, tinctures, alcoholic solutions or injection ampoules. The products are not necessarily made from a single ingredient. They can be formulated in combination with other TCM herbal products to provide additional benefits. Since Lingzhi is highly desirable for disease prevention, treatment for chronic ailments and improvement of general health and well-being, long-term application is generally recommended. Among the various Lingzhi preparations, products for oral use are generally the most convenient and economical. Thus, they are suited for the long-term applications. In contrast, injection ampoules are designed for special purposes and patients, and are more likely to cause side effects. They are not recommended for general use.

In making Lingzhi preparations, either fluidum extractum (the strength of 1ml of the concentrated liquid equals to 1g of the raw material) or extractum (the strength of 1g of the concentrated paste equals to 2–5g of the raw material) is to be obtained first. From the concentrates, various Lingzhi preparations are then made.

Preparation of Lingzhi fluidum extractum

Lingzhi contains polysaccharides, polypeptides, triterpenes, nucleoside, sterol, alkaloid, etc. The solubility of these components varies. For example, polysaccharides mainly dissolve in water, while triterpenes and sterol does in alcohol and organic solvents. Thus, to extract specific components, the appropriate solvent and method needs to be employed. Procedures for the extraction processes commonly used by the industry are briefly presented as follows.

Water extraction: Cut selected, dried Lingzhi fruiting bodies into dices or pieces. Place the cleaned and drained pieces in a steam-jacketed kettle with water filled to about 2/3 of the volume. Bring water to a boil, and cook for 3 hours. Drain and collect the extract from the kettle. To the pulp, add more water and repeat the boiling water extraction for another 3 hours. Filter and combine the extracts obtained from the two batches for concentration by heating under vacuum. Lingzhi fluidum extractum or extractum is thus made when the moisture content of resultant material reaches the pre-determined levels.

Alcohol extraction: Similar to the water extraction, food or drug grade 70% alcohol, instead of water, is used as the solvent in the alcohol extraction for Lingzhi. The amount of alcohol added should be enough to submerge the Lingzhi pieces. The kettle is equipped with a condenser to collect the alcohol vapor and turn it back into the liquid form for recycling. After 2 hours extraction, the extract is collected. Then, the same procedures are repeated twice using food or drug grade 70% and 60% alcohols for the 2nd and the 3rd batches, respectively. Combine all 3 extracts and allow it to settle for 24 hours. Collect the supernatant to be concentrated with heat under vacuum until a concentration of 1g Lingzhi/ml extract has been reached. To this initial concentrate, slowly add food or drug grade 95% alcohol while stirring until the alcohol content has reached 70%. After 24 hours or more, when the sedimentation is completed, collect the supernatant for another round of concentration with heat under vacuum. When the concentrate contains 2g Lingzhi/ml, with constant stirring, slowly add an equal amount of newly heated 70°C distilled water and preservative, if necessary. At 3-5°C , let the mixture stand for 24 hours or more to allow full sedimentation. By filtration, a clear solution is obtained. Heat the solution under vacuum to obtain the 2-5 g Lingzhi/ml concentration Lingzhi extractum.

Extraction by percolation: Clean and dry selected Lingzhi fruiting bodies. Grind them into granules of a size similar to a green bean.
Place the granules in a percolator approximately 2/3 of the total volume. Add food or drug grade 70% alcohol to a few centimeters above
submerge line for a 24 hours soaking with the percolator cover on. To
ensure a uniform extraction, weights may be placed on top of the fruiting body pieces. The flow rate applied for the percolation is generally
3–5 ml/min, based on 1000 g raw material. It can be adjusted according
to the actual amount. Alcohol may be replenished during the process
to avoid depletion of the solvent. Collect the initial 850 ml percolated
extract and continue to percolate till active components are exhausted.
In a distiller, concentrate the alcohol extract with heat under vacuum
until a thick paste is obtained. Meanwhile, the liquefied alcohol is collected through a condenser. Add the 850 ml extract collected earlier to
the extractum and mix well. Check the contents of alcohol and active
components in the mixture for quality assurance. For a Lingzhi fluidum
extractum, the concentration should be 1 g/ml; whereas, for an extractum, every gram should correspond to 2–5 g raw Lingzhi.

Combined alcohol and water extraction: In basically the same
manner as described above, Lingzhi raw material can also be extracted
by using alcohol followed by water on
the pulp, or vise versa, for the extraction.
The combined extract is then con cen-
trated to obtain either a fluidum extractum or extractum. Similarly, the liquid
culture medium and Lingzhi mycelium
collected from a submerged fermentation process can be made into these

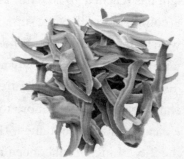

forms of the concentrates as well.

Cultivation of Lingzhi for its fruiting bodies

To a Lingzhi extractum, add starch or other filler. Mix well, screen Making of Lingzhi tablet productsture lower than 60℃ , cool, add magnesium stearate or other lubricants, and compress in mold to form tablets. In a sugar-coating device, plain tablets can be added with a coat of sugar to provide additional protection and convenience for use. The products should meet the standards specified under the Tablet Section in the Appendix of the *Chinese Pharmacopeia Part I* (2005 edition).

Making of Lingzhi capsule products

These products are made by filling capsules with the spray-dried powder obtained from a Lingzhi fluidum extractum or extractum. Due to the highly hygroscopic nature of the powder, moisture barrier property of the capsule and packaging material must be ensured, lest caking of the powder may occur.

To alleviate the caking problem, starch and/or other filler may be mixed in with the powder to form granules before capsule filling. Regardless of the format, the products must meet the standards set forth in the *Chinese Pharmacopeia Part I* that can be found in the Capsules Section in the Appendix of its 2005 edition.

Making of Lingzhi granular products

Lingzhi granular products can be used as is, or for instant drink applications. To make such products, dextrin and/or sugar are added to the fluidum extractum or extractum. After mixing, granules are made in a machine and sieved through a 12–14 mesh nylon cloth. Granules dried at a temperature below 60℃ are inspected before packaging. The moisture content and the size of the granules should meet the standards listed under the Granular Drugs Section in the Appendix of the *Chinese Pharmacopeia Part I* (2005 edition).

Making of Lingzhi syrup products

According to the dosage requirement, an appropriate amount of water is added to a fluidum extractum or extractum to yield a solution for further processing. Sugar syrup is prepared in advance for mixing with the abovementioned solution. The mixture, containing no less than 45g sugar/ml, is boiled, filtered, added with preservatives and adjusted to pH 3-3.5. The finished syrup, then, is checked for quality and filled in bottles. The product's quality should conform to all required standards specified in the Syrup Section in the Appendix of the *Chinese Pharmacopeia Part I* (2005 edition).

Making of Lingzhi tincture products

Generally, a 100 ml tincture should be equivalent to 20 g of Lingzhi. It can be prepared by the following methods:

(1) Dissolving/diluting method: Use sufficient amount of alcohol of a specified grade and concentration to dissolve and dilute the liquid Lingzhi concentrates. Allow the solution to stand and filter, if necessary, to obtain the tincture product with desired strength.

(2) Marinating method: Soak clean, dried Lingzhi fruiting body pieces in sufficient amount of 90% alcohol for 3-5 days. Collect the alcohol extract and re-soak the pulp in 75% alcohol for 1 day followed by soaking in 50% alcohol for another day. Distill the combined extract at a temperature below 70℃ under vacuum. Continue the distillation

till no smell of alcohol remains in the concentrate. Add required amount of freshly distilled water to the concentrate to arrive at a concentration of 20 g raw material/100 ml. The tincture product should be sealed and stored in a dark, cool place.

The products must meet the standards set forth in the *Chinese Pharmacopeia Part I* that can be found in the Tincture Section in the Appendix of its 2005 edition.

 ## Making of Lingzhi vinum

By immersing clean, dried Lingzhi fruiting body slices, dices or pieces in a liquor made from grains containing more than 50% of alcohol in a glass container, an alcoholic product can be made. In a dark room, marinate for 14 days at ambient temperature. Combine the supernatant from the marinade as well as the juice by squeezing the pulp, filter and add sugar or honey and/or caramel for coloring to obtain the final product. These products should establish criteria on alcohol and solids contents by the Vinum Section in the Appendix of the *Chinese Pharmacopeia Part I* (2005 edition).

 ## Manufacturing of Lingzhi injection ampoules

In 500 g of cleaned, dried and pulverized Lingzhi fruiting body, add 10 times of the amount of 95% alcohol. Soak for 24 hours at 60°C with constant stirring. Filter the mixture to obtain Filtrate A. To the pulp, 8 times of the amount of 85% alcohol is used for the soaking to get Filtrate B, followed by the addition of 6 times of the amount of 75% alcohol to the last pulp for getting Filtrate C. Combine Filtrates A, B and C, allow it to stand at 4–8°C overnight, filter and concentrate the filtrate in a distiller with heat under vacuum. By heating the alcohol-free concentrate in an evaporator or a steam-jacketed kettle, the moisture content is reduced as the total volume of the concentrate decrease to 1000 ml. Add 0.3% of the activated charcoal to the concentrate and heat at boiling temperature to remove pigments. With further filtration, a clear solution is obtained. After cooling, 0.2% Tween 80 is added followed by mixing and filtration. Blend in 1%–2% benzyl alcohol, adjust pH to about 6.5 and allow it to stand at 4–8℃ overnight. With filtrations to remove fine particles and microbes the solution is ready to be filled into ampoules and sealed for thermal sterilization. Quality of the injection products should meet all requirements specified in the Injection Section in the Appendix of the *Chinese Pharmacopeia Part I* (2005 edition).

To make injection ampoules from Lingzhi mycelium, the mycelia are dried and pulverized before boiling the raw material in water for 2 hours. Filtrates from 3 boiling water extractions are combined and concentrated. After cooling, add alcohol to reach 75% alcoholic content and allow it to stand for over 48 hours. Using a Bü chner funnel, the solution is filtered, while the alcohol is condensed and collected. By using 10% NaOH, the solution is adjusted to pH 8. After standing overnight in the ambient temperature, another sucking filtration is performed. Discard the sediments, adjust the solution's pH to 6 using a diluted sulfuric acid, and discard the sediments again. Add alcohol to the solution for an alcoholic content of 85%, and allow it to stand for 48 hours. On the solution at yet another sucking filtration, the alcohol is completely distilled. Then, 5% active carbon is added to the solution and the mixture is heated for 30 minutes. The mixture is subjected to a sucking filtration, and a preservative solution (i.e., 1% benzyl alcohol in 60℃ distilled water) is added to the filtrate with stirring. With distilled water added to volume, the solution is again filtered to remove fine particles followed by microbial removal by means of a refusion glass infundi-bulum. The filled ampoules are sealed and autoclaved to achieve sterilization for medical applications. Quality of the ampoules should meet all requirements specified in the Injection Section in the Appendix of the *Chinese Pharmacopeia Part I* (2005 edition).

Lingzhi spore powder can be used as the raw material for manufacturing products for injection applications as well. For the spore products, however, cell wall breaking is needed to facilitate the extraction of active components. The extraction and processing procedures similar to those employed for the fruiting body or mycelium are, nonetheless, necessary for the injection products made from the spores in order to meet the requirements by the stringent law and regulations.

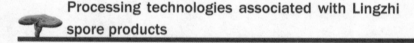

Processing technologies associated with Lingzhi spore products

Ganoderma spores as collected from the mature Lingzhi are fine powder. They can be sieved and cleaned prior to filling into gel capsules for administration. The lipid content of the spores can be extracted and made into soft-gel capsules as a more concentrated product. In order to facilitate the absorption, as well as the extraction, pre-treatment to break the cell-walls of the spores (sporoderms) may be applied.

Cell-wall breaking methodologies: Since the cell-wall of the spore is resistant to chemical and physical damages. It is, therefore, believed that by breaking the cell-walls, the bio-availability of the spore products can be improved. To break the cell-walls, mechanical, chemical and enzymatic methods have been tested and applied commercially. Due to the temperature and chemical sensitivities of the oil and active components, the applied methodology must not be too severe in order to protect the efficacy of the spore products. Consequently, the resultant improvement directly relates to the cell-wall breakage rate. Theoretically, the higher the rate, the more efficient is the absorption.

Supercritical fluid extraction (SFE): A recently available technology, SFE applies carbon dioxide under specific temperature and pressure to extract the unsaturated fatty acids and oil-soluble components, such as triterpenes, from the spores. Since carbon dioxide is a natural, non-toxic material and the conditions used for the extraction are milder than conventional solvent extraction, distillation or evaporation, spore oil products obtained by using SFE technology are believed to be pure and functionally active.

Appendix

Ganoderma (Lingzhi). *Chinese Pharmacopeia Part I*,
English edition, People's Medical Publishing House,
Beijing. 2005, 117-118.

Ganoderma is the dried sporophore of *Ganoderma lucidum* (Leyss. Ex Fr.) Karst. or *Ganoderma sinensis* Zhao,Xu et Zhang. (Fam. Polyporaceae). The drug is collected all the year, removed from foreign matter, attached rotten wood, sand or the lower stipe of the culture matrix, dried in the shade or stove an 40-50℃.

Description *Ganoderma lucidum* Outline firmbriate, pileus reniform, semi-rounded or subrounded, 10-18 cm in diameter, 1-2cm thick. Shell hard, yellowish-brown to reddish-brown, lustrous, with circular arrised stripe and radiate wrinkle, edge thin and even, frequently incurved slightly. The inner part white to brownish. Stip cylinder, laterally grown, few learning grown, 7-15 cm long, 1-3.5 cm in diameter, reddish-brown to purplish brown, luminous. Spore small and fine, yellowish-brown to purplish brown, luminous. Spore small and fine, yellow-brown. Odor, slightly aromatic, taste bitter and astringent.

Ganoderma sinensis Shell purplish-black, with lacquer-like luster. Sporophore rusty-brown. Stip 17-23 cm long.

Cultivated Ganoderma Sporophore relatively sturdy, plump,1-22 cm in diameter, 1.5-4cm thick. Shell frequently coated with a large

of
yellowish-brown powder-like spores.

Identification　　(1)Powder: pale brown, dark brown, yellowish-brown, slim, slightly curved, branched, 2.5–6.5cm in diameter. Spores brown, ovate apex even, external walls colourless, inner walls with protuberance, 8–12cm long, 5–8cm wide.

(2)To 2 g of the coarse powder add 30 ml of methanol, heat and reflux for 30 minutes, filter, evaporate the filtrate to dryness, add 2ml of methanol to dissolve the residue, and use it as the test solution.Prepare a solution of Ganoderma reference drug in the same manner, and use it as the reference drug solution. Carry out the method for thin layer chromatography(Appendix VI B), using silica gel G as the coating substance and mixture of petroleum ether (60–90℃) ethyl formate and formic acid(15:5:1, upper layer) as the mobile phase. Apply separately to the plate 4ml each of the two solutions. After developing and removal of the plate, dry in air, examine under ultraviolet light at 365nm. The fluorescent spot in the chromatogram obtained with the test solution corresponds in position and colour to the spot in the chromatogram obtained with the reference drug solution.

Water　　Carry out the method for determination of water (Appendix IX H, method 1), not more than 17.0 percent.

Total ash　　Not more than 0.5 percent(Appendix IX K).

Acid-insoluble ash　　Not more than 0.5 percent (Appendix IX K).

Extractives　　Carry out the hot extraction method for determine of water-solution extractives (Appendix X A), not less than 3.0 percent.

Assay　　*Reference solution* Weigh accurately a quantity of anhydrous dextrose CRS, dried previously to constant weigh at 105℃, in a volumetric flask, dissolve and dilute with water to volume, and mix well to produce a solution containing 0.1 mg per ml as the reference solution.

Calibration standard Measure accurately 0.2, 0.4, 0.8, 1.0 and 1.2ml of the reference solution respectively into a 10ml stopper test tube and add to a total of 2.0ml with water, Measure accurately 6ml of the solution of anthrone sulphate (dissolve 0.1 g of anthrone, accurately weighed, to 100ml of 80% sulfuric acid, and mix well), mix well, heat on a water bath for 15 minutes, cool on an ice water bath for 15 minutes. Carry out the method for ultraviolet spectrophotometry and colourimetry (Appendix V A), perform a black determination with the relative test solution, measure the absorbance at 625 nm and plot the standard curve, using the absorbance as ordinate and the concentration as abscissa.

Test solution Weigh accurately 2 g of the powder into a Soxhlet's extractor, extract with 90 ml of water under reflux on an electric heated thermostat until the extract colourless, transfer the extract to a 100ml volumetric flask, dilute with water to volume, and mix well. Measure accurately 10ml , add 150 ml of ethanol and mix well, cool at 4°C for 12 hours, removal of the flask, centrifuge, and discard the upper layer of the clarified liquid. Dissolve the residue with water and transfer it to 50 ml volumetric flask, dilute with water to volume, and mix well.

Procedure Measure accurately 2ml of the test solution, into a 10ml stopper test tube, carry out the procedure as described under calibration standard, beginning at the words "measure accurately 6 ml of···", measure the absorbance at 625 nm and read out the weight of anhydrous dextrose (mg) in the test solution from the standard curve, and calculate the content of polysaccharides of Ganoderma.

It contains not less than 0.50 percent of polysaccharides of Ganoderma, calculated as anhydrous dextrose ($C_6H_{12}O_6$) with reference to the dried drug.

Action   To replenish *qi* and ease the mind, relieve cough and asthma.

Indications   Dizziness, insomnia, palpitation, shortness of breath, asthenic cough and asthma.

Usage and dosage   6–12g.

Storage   Preserve in a dry place, protected from mould and moth

图书在版编目(CIP)数据

灵芝　从神奇到科学=Lingzhi　From Mystery to Science:　英文/林志彬编著.–北京:北京大学医学出版社,2009
ISBN　978-7-81116-828-0

Ⅰ.灵…　Ⅱ.林…　Ⅲ.灵芝–基本知识—英文Ⅳ.R282.71

中国版本图书馆 CIP 数据核字(2009)第 094630 号

灵芝　从神奇到科学

Lingzhi　From Mystery to Science

编　　著：	林志彬	
	Zhi–Bin Lin	
出版发行：	北京大学医学出版社(电话:010–82802230)	
地　　址：	(100191)北京市海淀区学院路 38 号　北京大学医学部院内	
网　　址：	http://www.pumpress.com.cn	
E–　mail：	booksale@bjmu.edu.cn	
印　　刷：	北京圣彩虹制版印刷技术有限公司	
经　　销：	新华书店	
责任编辑：	冯智勇	
版式设计：	朱靓　殷花	封面设计：　殷花
责任校对：	何力	责任印制：　张京生
开　　本：	880mm×1230mm　1/32　印张：　6　字数：　135 千字	
版　　次：	2009 年 6 月第 1 版,2009 年 6 月第 1 次印刷	
书　　号：	ISBN　978-7-81116-828-0	
定　　价：	38.00 元